Pain Management for Advanced Practice

Multimodal Approaches

Pain Management for Advanced Practice

Multimodal Approaches

Angela Starkweather, PhD, ACNP-BC, CNRN, FAAN
Professor, Center for Advancement in Managing Pain
University of Connecticut School of Nursing
Storrs, Connecticut

Paula S. McCauley, DNP, APRN, ACNP-BC, FAANP
Acute Care Nurse Practitioner, Cardiology, Cardiothoracic Surgery
University of Connecticut Health
Farmington, Connecticut
Associate Professor
University of Connecticut School of Nursing
Storrs, Connecticut

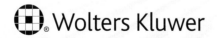 Wolters Kluwer

Philadelphia • Baltimore • New York • London
Buenos Aires • Hong Kong • Sydney • Tokyo

Acquisitions Editor: Nicole Dernoski
Product Development Editor: Tom Conville
Editorial Coordinator: Jeremiah Kiely
Marketing Manager: Linda Wetmore
Production Project Manager: Sadie Buckallew
Design Coordinator: Joseph Clark
Manufacturing Coordinator: Kathleen Brown
Prepress Vendor: S4Carlisle Publishing Services

9 8 7 6 5 4 3 2 1

Printed in China.

Library of Congress Cataloging-in-Publication Data

ISBN-13: 978-1-975103-35-4

ISBN-10: 1-975103-35-1

Library of Congress Control Number: 2019910750

RRS1908

I dedicate this text to all of the patients and families who are affected by pain, as you were the inspiration; and to my dear children who are the light of my life.
—ANGELA STARKWEATHER

I dedicate this text to the providers who will care for those patients and families impacted by pain; and to my husband Jim for his unending support and love.
—PAULA MCCAULEY

ACKNOWLEDGMENTS

T hank you to our patients and families who have taught us so much about how to manage pain, to the contributors who continue to give them hope every day, and to all the clinicians who are working endlessly to provide safe and effective care to people who are suffering.

PREFACE

P ain management is a crucial aspect of patient care that every advanced practice clinician should feel comfortable administering. However, the opioid epidemic has caused a lot of fear in both patients and clinicians, with the unfortunate result of making it more difficult to receive safe and effective multimodal care. This text provides information on pharmacologic and nonpharmacologic pain management strategies with highlights on evidence-based decision making and integration of attending to the biopsychosocial and spiritual being across acute and chronic pain conditions. We hope that this text is helpful as you continue to care for the patients and families who live with pain.

Approaches to pain management included in this text:

- Physical examination and diagnostic testing
- Cognitive behavioral therapy
- Yoga, massage, and acupuncture
- Analgesics and adjunctive pharmacologic agents
- Invasive pain interventions
- Treatment of pain in the addicted patient
- System-level pain management

Special features include key points that are included in each chapter and case studies when appropriate for direct application of the content.

CONTRIBUTOR LIST

Moorice Caparó, MD
Resident Physician
Department of Physical Medicine and
  Rehabilitation
Harvard Medical School
Boston, Massachusetts

Edward Gillis, MD
Resident Physician
Department of Radiology
University of Connecticut Health Center
Farmington, Connecticut

Jessica W. Guite, PhD
Associate Professor
Pediatrics & Center for Advancement
  in Managing Pain (CAMP)
School of Medicine & School of
  Nursing
University of Connecticut
Storrs, Connecticut
Pediatric Psychologist & Research
  Scientist
Center for Behavioral Health
Connecticut Children's Medical
  Center (CCMC)
Hartford, Connecticut

Seth Hagymasi, PT, DPT, OCS, FAAOMPT
Supervisor, Spine Rehabilitation
Department of Rehabilitation
UConn Health
Farmington, Connecticut

Thomas M. Julian, BA, BSN, RN
Research Assistant, PhD Candidate
Center for Advancement in Managing
  Pain
School of Nursing
University of Connecticut
Storrs, Connecticut

Kyounghae Kim, PhD, RN, NP-C
Assistant professor
School of Nursing
University of Connecticut
Storrs, Connecticut
Advanced Practice Registered Nurse
UConn Musculoskeletal Institute
University of Connecticut Health Center
Farmington, Connecticut

Paula S. McCauley, DNP, APRN, ACNP-BC, FAANP
Acute Care Nurse Practitioner,
  Cardiology, Cardiothoracic Surgery
University of Connecticut Health
Farmington, Connecticut
Associate Professor
University of Connecticut School of
  Nursing
Storrs, Connecticut

Deborah Dillon McDonald, PhD, RN
Associate Professor
School of Nursing
University of Connecticut
Storrs, Connecticut

Mallory Perry, PhD, RN
Adjunct Faculty
School of Nursing
University of Connecticut
Storrs, Connecticut
Clinical Nurse II
Pediatric Intensive Care Unit
Connecticut Children's Medical Center
Hartford, Connecticut

Trinh Pham, PharmD, BCOP
Clinical Specialist, Oncology Pharmacy
  Services
Quality Improvement and Performance
  Management
Yale New Haven Health, Smilow Cancer
  Hospital
New Haven, Connecticut

Michael Reiss, PsyD
Assistant Clinical Professor
Department of Pediatrics
School of Medicine
University of Connecticut
Storrs, Connecticut
Pediatric Psychologist
Weight Management Program
Connecticut Children's Medical Center
  (CCMC)
Hartford, Connecticut

Charan Singh, MBBS, MD
Assistant Professor
Department of Interventional Radiology
UConn Health
Farmington, Connecticut

**Angela Starkweather, PhD, ACNP-BC,
  CNRN, FAAN**
Professor and Associate Dean for Academic
  Affairs
School of Nursing, Center for Advancement
  in Managing Pain
School of Medicine, Genetics and Genome
  Sciences
University of Connecticut
Storrs, Connecticut

Jonathan Sylvain, PT, DPT, OCS, FAAOMPT
Spine Clinical Rehab Program Manager
Hartford Healthcare Rehabilitation
  Network
Hartford Healthcare
Farmington, Connecticut

Miguel Ernesto Velez, MD
Resident Physician
Department of Physical Medicine and
  Rehabilitation
Harvard Medical School
Boston, Massachusetts

Joseph Walker, MD
Assistant Professor
Orthopedic Surgery and Neurosurgery
University of Connecticut School of
  Medicine
Farmington, Connecticut
Faculty Staff
UConn Musculoskeletal Institute
  Comprehensive Spine Center
University of Connecticut Health Center
Farmington, Connecticut

CONTENTS

CHAPTER 1

BIOPSYCHOSOCIAL MODEL OF PAIN AND PATIENT-CENTERED PAIN MANAGEMENT

Angela Starkweather

Definition and Epidemiology of Pain

Pain has been described throughout time as a symptom, similar to fatigue or depression, that is capable of overwhelming a person's normal capacity to cope and function, in which case it can become a health condition in and of itself. The International Association for the Study of Pain (1994) defines pain as "an unpleasant sensory and emotional experience associated with actual or potential tissue damage or described in terms of such damage" (p. 1). This definition describes pain as a complex phenomenon with multiple components that impact a person's psychosocial and physical functioning. Another clinical definition of pain, which was proposed by McCaffery (1968), states, "Pain is whatever the experiencing person says it is, existing whenever he says it does" (p. 8). This definition is accepted worldwide and reinforces that pain is a highly personal and subjective experience, a reason that all accepted guidelines consider the patient's report to be the most reliable indicator of pain. Although both definitions refer to the individual's report of pain, some people are unable to communicate because of developmental or cognitive status, disability, disease, or mechanical obstruction. In these situations, we must rely on behavioral cues, facial expressions, or other modalities to identify pain.

Pain is one of the most common reasons for seeking medical care across all age groups and is often a presenting symptom of an underlying injury or pathology (National Institutes of Health, 2016). It can serve as an indicator of disease severity, an index of prognosis, and a determinant of health. The prevalence of chronic pain in the general population of U.S. adults has been shown to exceed 48% in some studies, with low back and neck pain, osteoarthritis, and headache being the most common (National Academies, 2011). Reportedly 25.3 million American adults suffer from daily pain and 14.4 million experience severe pain (Nahin, 2015). It is currently estimated that pain costs Americans $635 billion annually for direct and indirect care, and lost productivity (National Academies, 2011).

One in four children have episodes of chronic pain that last 3 months or longer (King et al., 2011; Korterink, Diederen, Benninga, & Tabbers, 2015). Similar to adult populations, the prevalence of chronic pain is higher in girls compared with boys and increases with age (pubertal development). The median prevalence of idiopathic pain in community-based samples of children ranges from 11% to 38%, with the most common chronic pain conditions being reported in up to 51% for headache, 41.2% for abdominal pain, up to 40% for musculoskeletal pain, and 24% for low back pain (Brun Sundblad, Saartok, & Engström, 2007; Korterink et al., 2015; McBeth & Jones, 2007). Chronic pain is associated with significant psychosocial and physical burden for children and families and ranks among the costliest health conditions in the United States, at an estimated $19.5 billion per year (Groenewald, Essner, Wright, Fesinmeyer, & Palermo, 2014). Effective multimodal treatment for pain in children entails efforts to reduce pain severity, non interference with daily activities, and preservation of physical, psychological, social, and role functions. A major goal is to prevent immediate and future disability because there is convincing evidence that childhood pain predisposes an individual for pain chronicity and development of comorbid pain disorders in adulthood (Walker, Dengler-Crish, Rippel, & Bruehl, 2010).

Nociception and Pain

The physiologic systems that result in pain developed, from an evolutionary standpoint, as a protective mechanism to alert the individual of actual or potential tissue injury, and it typically resolves with the normal phases of healing. When pain continues beyond normal healing and becomes chronic, it no longer serves any useful purpose and is referred to as pathologic pain. Although the physiologic mechanisms that contribute to the transition from acute to chronic pain are not completely understood at this time, there are several lines of evidence suggesting that the severity, impact, and resolution of pain may be influenced by genetics. First we will discuss the physiology of pain as a protective factor and then possible alterations that can lead to chronic pain.

> ▶ **KEY POINT**
>
> Many pharmacologic agents target the substances released in response to injury. For instance, prostaglandin inhibitors, such as nonsteroidal anti-inflammatory drugs, prevent prostaglandin production by inhibiting the action of an enzyme, cyclooxygenase, that is used to form prostaglandins. Other pharmacologic agents work centrally, in the central nervous system (CNS), to increase or inhibit substances released along the nociceptive pathway.

The cells that are capable of transducing and transmitting noxious pain signals are known as nociceptors, and they are found in the skin, muscle, connective tissue, circulatory system, and the viscera of the abdomen, pelvis, and thorax. Nociceptors are free nerve endings that transduce noxious stimuli, which can be mechanical, thermal, or chemical, into neuronal action potentials that are transmitted centrally to the spinal cord and brain. Stimulation of nociceptors can be the result of direct nerve damage, exposure to noxious stimuli at a specific threshold, and the release of chemicals at the site of injury. During tissue injury, a host of inflammatory mediators are activated to travel to the site of injury. Inflammatory mediators, as well as chemical mediators released in response to the injury (K^+, H^+, lactate, histamine, serotonin, bradykinins, and prostaglandins), alter the membrane potential of nociceptors, thereby facilitating depolarization and generation of action potentials.

The mechanisms that lead to the perception of nociceptive pain are described as transduction, transmission, perception, and modulation (Figure 1-1). This normal response of the somatosensory system to noxious stimuli is the process known as nociception. When the brain receives and interprets the information as an unpleasant painful sensation, it is known as nociceptive pain (Haines, 2012). This exquisite network of cells, fibers, and nociceptive pathways can result in pain only when the brain is capable of receiving and interpreting stimuli. However, the activity of the nociceptive system does not always result in the experience of pain; thus, pain and nociception are

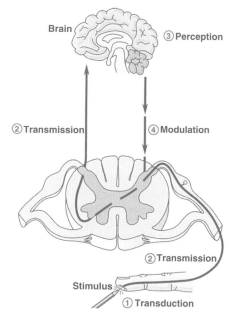

Figure 1-1. Processes of pain signaling.

not synonymous. The brain has a powerful influence on how we perceive sensory information and may filter or block pain information from awareness or change our perception of the sensory information (Pasero & Portenoy, 2011). This is an important concept for some of the pharmacologic and nonpharmacologic therapies used to manage pain, such as distraction, guided imagery, or cognitive behavioral therapy (CBT).

Transduction

Tissue damage results in the release of chemical mediators from damaged cells that activate nociceptors. These chemical mediators include prostaglandins, bradykinin, serotonin, substance P, and histamine (Starkweather & Pair, 2013). When the chemical mediators attach to the membrane of the nociceptor, it can result in the opening of sodium channels, which activate the nociceptor and cause the generation of an action potential, an electrical impulse.

Transmission

The action potential subsequently moves from the site of nociceptor activation along specialized afferent nerve fibers that carry pain impulses, known as A-delta and C fibers, to the spinal cord. A-delta fibers are thinly myelinated sensory fibers that send pain impulses faster than unmyelinated C fibers. Because of the myelin covering the A-delta fibers, they are capable of transmitting sharp, stabbing pain sensations, whereas C fibers transmit aching, burning-type pain sensations. Substance P and other neurotransmitters allow the action potential to proceed across the cleft to the dorsal horn of the spinal cord, where it ascends the spinothalamic tract to the thalamus and midbrain.

█ Perception

Fibers from the thalamus send the nociceptive message to the somatosensory cortex, frontal and parietal lobes as well as the limbic system, where pain is perceived and interpreted on the basis of past experience, beliefs, attitudes, and meaning.

█ Modulation

Activation of the midbrain results in the release of substances such as endorphins, enkephalins, serotonin, and dynorphin from neurons that descend to the lower areas of the brain and spinal cord, stimulating the release of endogenous opioids that inhibit transmission of pain impulses at the dorsal horn.

Once the pain signal is transmitted to the cell bodies of pain neurons in the dorsal root ganglion, they enter the dorsal horn of the spinal cord by way of the posterior nerve roots, where the A-delta and C fibers synapse with interneurons, anterior motor neurons, and sympathetic preganglionic neurons. A specific area of the spinal cord (referred to as laminae II and III regions) known as the substantia gelatinosa houses multiple synaptic connections among the primary sensory afferent neurons, interneurons, and anterolateral ascending fibers (Figure 1-2). This region is important because pain signal transmission can be modulated by CNS activity or release of endogenous substances. Lamina V of the spinal cord receives somatic input from mechanical, thermal, and chemical receptors, besides visceral receptors, which is thought to explain the potential for referred pain, when pain from a visceral organ is perceived at the body surface.

Synaptic transmission in the spinal cord is carried out by a number of neurotransmitters and neuropeptides, such as substance P, glutamate, γ-aminobutyric acid, cholecystokinin, and calcitonin gene–related peptide, by binding to the next neuron in the pathway and generating action potentials. Spinal interneurons conduct pain signals across the spinal segment and carry them to the brain by way of the ascending spinal pathways, mainly the anterolateral (aka spinothalamic) tract.

Pain impulses enter the brainstem reticular activating formation, thalamus, and lower brain centers, causing conscious perception of pain. Neurons in the rostral pons secrete norepinephrine, which has an analgesic

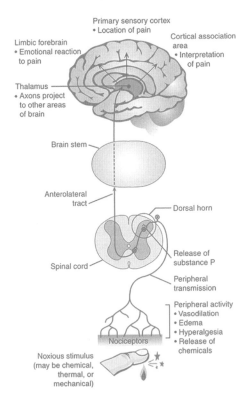

Figure 1-2. Anterolateral nociceptive pathways travel up the spinal cord and project to the thalamus, somatosensory cortex, cortical association areas, and limbic structures.

effect, and continue on to the raphe magnus. Conduction of pain signals to the periaqueductal gray in the midbrain, which has a high concentration of endogenous opioids, is also sent to the raphe magnus through release of 5-hydroxytryptamine and serotonin. Descending pathways from the brain can either facilitate or inhibit ascending pain impulses or the interpretation of pain.

Description of Pain

Many terms are used to describe pain, and this can be informative in discerning the primary source of pain. Localized pain is easily identified by the patient and is located in a confined area. The clinician can ask the patient to point to the area of pain in order to ascertain whether it is localized or not. In cases of generalized pain, the patient will report many areas that do not follow dermatologic patterns (described later). Somatic pain refers to pain that originates from the peripheral or spinal nerves, whereas visceral pain arises from the internal organs of the body. Affective-motivational pain is strongly modulated by context and cognitive appraisal of pain and may include descriptions of frustration, anger, hopelessness, and helplessness. Sensory aspects of pain mainly focus on the intensity of pain, with terms such as sharp/dull, shooting, or lancinating. The pain descriptors used by the patient are important for the clinician in identifying a potential source of the pain and comorbidities (e.g., anxiety and depression) that may be accompanying the pain experience.

Nociceptor pathways are maintained in a specific anatomic order in the spinal cord and somatosensory cortex of the brain. Therefore, when pain originates from peripheral afferent nerves, the brain is able to localize pain to a specific region of the body. The anatomic map of each spinal nerve travels down a specific area of the body, which is referred to as a sensory dermatome (Figure 1-3). When a spinal nerve is exposed to compression or direct damage, it can cause the characteristic sensations of tingling and burning that follows a specific dermatomal pattern. This form of pain is called a radiculopathy and commonly occurs with spinal compression because of a herniated disk or postherpetic neuralgia. Other types of pain do not follow a dermatomal pattern, such as diabetic neuropathy, which characteristically affects the distal extremities in a stocking- or glove-like pattern. Pain that is caused by a lesion or disease affecting the somatosensory system is termed neuropathic pain.

Chronic widespread pain, including fibromyalgia, is considered to be an extreme example of centralized pain, as patients describe multiple sites of pain outside of normal dermatomal patterns (Arnold et al., 2016). Individuals with fibromyalgia report diffuse hyperalgesia (increased pain to normally painful stimuli) and allodynia (pain to normally nonpainful stimuli). These are key clinical features of neuropathic pain; however, the fact that they do not align with the somatosensory map of the brain or peripheral nerves in chronic widespread pain suggests a fundamental problem with augmented pain or sensory processing in the CNS (Clauw, 2014). Centralized pain can play a role in nociceptive and neuropathic pain; however, as alterations in the neural networks of the CNS become established as "memories," the centralization of pain becomes more prominent (Figure 1-4). These pain memories have been documented through functional magnetic imaging studies that have shown different

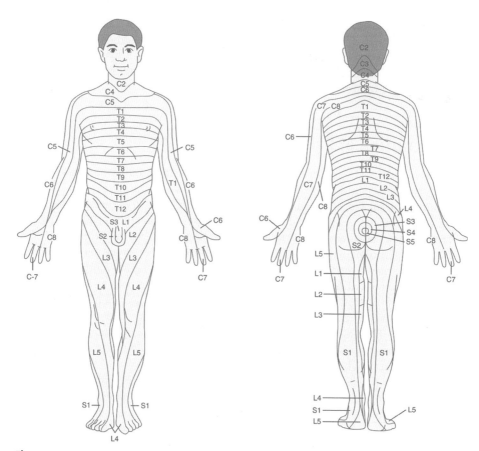

Figure 1-3. Sensory dermatomes.

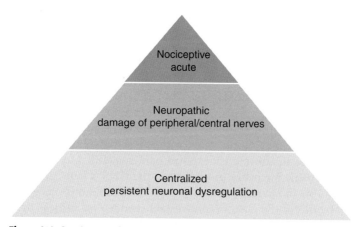

Figure 1-4. Continuum of pain processing.

areas of the brain involved in processing pain when comparing patients suffering from acute and localized pain with those suffering from chronic and diffuse pain.

Thus, even when centralized pain is a component of nociceptive pain, it resolves along with the acute pain. As a component of neuropathic pain, centralized pain causes characteristic symptoms of hyperalgesia and allodynia and may also contribute to radiating, spreading, or mirror-image pain (Jancalek, 2011). As a prototype of centralized pain, fibromyalgia is an example of how pain may arise without any observable lesion of the peripheral or central nerves but arises because of the perturbations in peripheral and central processing and/or deficient descending pain inhibition.

Biopsychosocial Model of Pain

The sensory and affective components of pain call for a multimodal treatment strategy that holistically addresses the needs of the patient and family—biologic, psychological, social, and spiritual (McCaffery, Herr, & Pasero, 2011). One of the most widely accepted models for guiding chronic pain management, the biopsychosocial model of pain (Figure 1-5), provides a framework for understanding the interactions among biologic, psychological, and sociocultural factors that influence the impact of pain on the individual (Gatchel, Peng, Peters, Fuchs, & Turk, 2007). A basic premise of the model is the distinction between pain as disease and pain as illness. Disease represents the pathophysiologic process of nociception whether it is through tissue injury, a neural lesion, or other source, whereas illness refers to the subjective

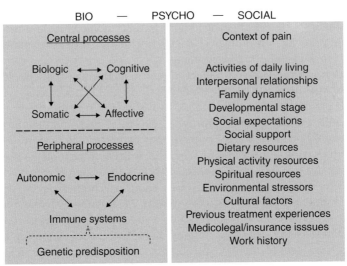

Figure 1-5. Biopsychosocial model of pain. Modified from Gatchel, R. J. (2004). Comorbidity of chronic mental and physical health conditions: The biopsychosocial perspective. *American Psychologist, 59*, 792–805. Copyright © 2004. Adapted with permission of the American Psychological Association.

experience of pain and its impact on individual functioning. Nociceptive input is filtered through an individual's biologic (anatomic, physiologic, genetic) architecture, psychological status, and sociocultural context, with each of these factors contributing to how the individual lives with and responds to the perception of pain (illness).

Much of our knowledge about the mechanisms contributing to pain has been focused on the social aspects because they are more easily accessible in terms of measurement. However, with the era of genomics, we have learned much about genetic predisposition to chronic pain conditions, and this area of science is just beginning to provide explanations on why some people are more prone to having disabling pain. Other biologic and psychological aspects of pain are also being explored in terms of their influence on pain outcomes. For instance, it is well known that anxiety and depression can amplify pain. Recent research in pain catastrophizing, the view of having the worst possible outcome, as well as sleep disturbances has shown that these aspects can heavily influence how a person experiences pain. Taken together, it is important to assess all of these aspects of the patient in order to provide an optimal situation in which the patient can develop effective coping strategies and identify therapeutic targets to mitigate the deleterious consequences of pain.

Pain Management

In order to identify effective pain management strategies, clinicians work from the history and physical assessment, results from laboratory and diagnostic testing, as well as patient preferences to determine the best approach. An additional component in the matrix is the patient's expectations of what they will experience, what they will receive, and how quickly they will be alleviated from pain. It is critical to communicate the role of the patient and family in the process of pain management and stress the importance of engaged goal-setting, monitoring, and motivation in each domain (biologic, psychological, social, spiritual) in order to experience significant results in pain and overall well-being.

Education is a fundamental aspect of pain management that should entail information about the condition, treatment options, and expectations, and it ideally involves the patient and family members. Providing information about how the patient and family can self-manage improves their self-efficacy and their own ability to effectively manage pain on a daily basis. It may be performed one on one, in group sessions with or without peer mentors, or with written or technologic resources.

Treating the psychological aspects of the pain experience may entail CBT, an evidence-based approach that involves using psychotherapeutic strategies to help solve problems and teach skills to modify dysfunctional thinking and behavior. Specific types of CBT have been studied in chronic pain populations, including mindfulness-based cognitive therapy, acceptance and commitment therapy, and compassion-focused therapy. To address kinesiophobia, or the fear of movement, patients may need referrals to physical therapy or rehabilitation specialists. Problem-solving deficiencies have been shown in patients with chronic pain, and healthcare providers can use various strategies to assist the patient and family to learn how to problem-solve.

As patients learn effective skills to help manage their pain, they may require the means to monitor their condition, which can be done through journaling, in written, electronic, or online formats. Goal-setting is an important part of this process, which should take place mutually between the patient and the healthcare team. Goals should entail functional outcomes that the patient can strive for and are written in the SMART format:

Specific (simple, sensible, significant)
Measurable (meaningful, motivating)
Achievable (agreed, attainable)
Relevant (reasonable, realistic, resourced, and results-based)
Time-limited (set a date for evaluation and modification)

The social aspects of pain management may involve reducing periods of isolation, identifying peer support groups, and accessing community and work-related resources for managing pain. Social determinants of health can play a significant role in creating barriers for the individual with chronic pain, including such things as lack of family support, education, and financial means to access healthcare providers. Identifying resources that the patient population can access in order to meet goals in physical activity and diet may involve partnership with community centers and social services.

Learning new skills in pain self-management, including goal-setting, monitoring, and self-regulation, can provide new avenues for the patient and family to modify learned behaviors and establish new neural pathways in their response to pain. Skills such as mindfulness meditation, guided imagery, therapeutic breathing, and sleep hygiene can lead to physiologic changes along the pain neuroaxis that either decrease pain-inducing molecules (such as substance P) or increase endogenous enkephalins that inhibit pain signaling (Figure 1-6).

The use of analgesics for mitigating acute pain is well described and will be covered in a later chapter. The World Health Organization's analgesic ladder is one of the most frequently cited resources for managing medications for pain. Although analgesics offer an important strategy for managing pain, their long-term use has led to a wide range of iatrogenic health conditions and has spurred the ongoing opioid epidemic. Use of long-term analgesics in specific populations who are carefully monitored for adverse effects and outcomes is undoubtedly an ethical approach for those unable to function without analgesics.

Although more research is needed to understand the progression from acute to chronic pain, it is clear that the limited, siloed strategies of the prevalent pain management system have not addressed the scope of pain in America. The National Institutes of Health National Pain Strategy (2016); the National Academies of Sciences, Engineering, and Medicine (2017); the Centers for Disease Control and Prevention opioid guidelines (Dowell, Haegerich, & Chou, 2016); the updated pain mandate from the Joint Commission (2017); the Food and Drug Administration (2017); and the American College of Physicians Clinical Practice Guidelines (Qaseem, Wilt, McLean, Forciea, & Clinical Guidelines Committee of the American College of Physicians, 2017) recommend evidence-informed, comprehensive pain care while conceding that past strategies generally, and the use of opioid medications

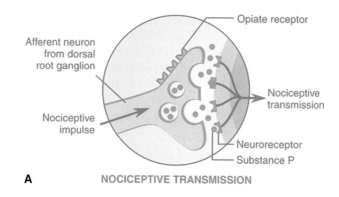

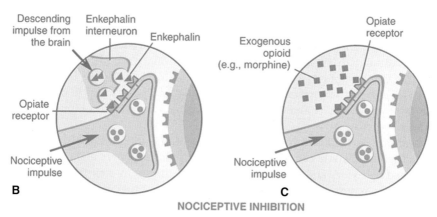

Figure 1-6. Pain transmission and inhibition at the molecular level. A, Nociceptive transmission to higher levels of the central nervous system. B, Nociception inhibited through binding of endogenous opioids (e.g., enkephalin). The release of substance P is prevented. C, Nociception inhibited through binding of exogenous opioid (e.g., morphine). Release of substance P is prevented.

specifically, have not remedied but rather exacerbated chronic pain, abuse, addiction, illness behavior, and disability.

Patient-Centered Pain Management

Patient-centered care prioritizes patient preferences, needs, desires, and experiences as part of the healthcare experience instead of the traditional paternalistic, provider-centric, and disease-driven approach (McComack & McCane, 2017). By recognizing the unique context that the patient brings to the experience, healthcare providers can empower patients and families to take a more active role in their health and well-being by partnering with them to better meet their goals. This may entail assisting the patient and family to set realistic goals and problem-solve some of the barriers they perceive in being able to reach their goals, as well as identifying resources that may serve as facilitators toward engaging in behaviors that will help them reach the state of health that they have set out to achieve (Newton-John, Mason, & Hunter, 2014).

Patients and families often come to healthcare providers with many preconceptions about pain management as being able to provide an immediate fix to their problem. However, effective pain management often requires behavioral changes that are challenging, such as changing sedentary habits into more active lifestyles and eating low-fat foods that are less inflammatogenic, and therefore less likely to contribute to the immune-related dysregulation that characterizes chronic pain. Throughout the process of identifying areas for behavioral change, the patient should be regarded as the expert in terms of knowing how they can best achieve the changes required, resources they may require, and adjunctive tools that will help them apply the behaviors in their daily life (Phillips et al., 2014). Our role as healthcare providers is not to tell patients what to do and how to do it, but to provide the best options on the basis of evidence and identify resources to assist them in building skills of resilience and ways to empower their own capabilities to achieve their goals toward relieving pain, improving function, and maintaining hope throughout their journey.

REFERENCES

Arnold, L. M., Choy, E., Clauw, D. J., Goldenberg, D. L., Haris, R. E., Helfenstein, M., Jr., . . . Wang, G. (2016). Fibromyalgia and chronic pain syndromes: A white paper detailing current challenges in the field. *Clinical Journal of Pain, 32*(9), 737–746.

Brun Sundblad, G. M., Saartok, T., & Engström, L. M. (2007). Prevalence and co-occurrence of self-rated pain and perceived health in school-children: Age and gender differences. *European Journal of Pain, 11*(2), 171–180.

Clauw, D. J. (2014). Fibromyalgia: A clinical review. *JAMA, 311*, 1547–1555.

Dowell, D., Haegerich, T. M., & Chou, R. (2016). CDC guideline for prescribing opioids for chronic pain—United States, 2016. *MMWR Recommendations and Reports, 65*(1), 1–49.

Food and Drug Administration. (2017). *FDA education blueprint for health care providers involved in the management or support of patients with pain.* Washington, DC: Author.

Gatchel, R. J., Peng, Y. B., Peters, M. L., Fuchs, P. N., & Turk, D. C. (2007). The biopsychosocial approach to chronic pain: Scientific advances and future directions. *Psychological Bulletin, 133*, 581–624.

Groenewald, C. B., Essner, B. S., Wright, D., Fesinmeyer, M. D., & Palermo, T. M. (2014). The economic costs of chronic pain among a cohort of treatment-seeking adolescents in the United States. *Journal of Pain, 15*(9), 925–933.

Haines, D. E. (2012). *Fundamental neuroscience for basic and clinical applications* (4th ed.). New York, NY: Saunders.

International Association for the Study of Pain. (1994). Part III: Pain terms, a current list with definitions and notes on usage. In H. Merseky & N. Bogduk (Eds.), *Classification of chronic pain* (2nd ed., pp. 209–214). Seattle, WA: Author.

Jancalek, R. (2011). Signaling mechanisms in mirror image pain pathogenesis. *Annals of Neurosciences, 18*(3), 123–127.

Joint Commission. (2017). *Joint Commission enhances pain assessment and management requirements for accredited hospitals.* Washington, DC: Author.

King, S., Chambers, C. T., Huguet, A., MacNevin, R. C., McGrath, P. J., Parker, L., & MacDonald, A. J. (2011). The epidemiology of chronic pain in children and adolescents revisited: A systematic review. *Pain, 152*, 2729–2738.

Korterink, J. J., Diederen, K., Benninga, M. A., & Tabbers, M. M. (2015). Epidemiology of pediatric functional abdominal pain disorders: A meta-analysis. *PLoS One, 10*(5), e0126982.

McCaffery, M. (1968). *Nursing practice theories related to cognition, bodily pain, and man-environment interactions.* Los Angeles: University of California.

McBeth, J., & Jones, K. (2007). Epidemiology of chronic musculoskeletal pain. *Best Practice & Research. Clinical Rheumatology, 21*(3), 403-425. http://dx.doi.org/10.1016/j.berh.2007.03.003

McCaffery, M., Herr, K., & Pasero, C. (2011). Assessment. In C. Pasero & M. McCaffery (Eds.), *Pain assessment and pharmacologic management* (pp. 13–176). St Louis, MO: Mosby/Elsevier.

McComack, B., & McCane, T. (2017). *Person-centered practice in nursing and health care.* Chichester, UK: Wiley Blackwell.

Nahin, R. L. (2015). Estimates of pain prevalence and severity in adults: United States, 2012. *Journal of Pain, 16*(8), 769–780.

National Academies, Institute of Medicine (2011). Relieving pain in America: A blueprint for transforming prevention, care, education and research. Washington, D.C.: National Academies Press.

National Academies of Sciences, Engineering, and Medicine. (2017). *Consensus study report highlights. Pain management and the opioid epidemic: Balancing societal and individual benefits and risks of prescription opioid use.* Washington, DC: National Academies Press.

National Institutes of Health. (2016). *National pain strategy, a comprehensive population health-level strategy for pain.* Washington, DC: Department of Health and Human Services.

Newton-John, T. R., Mason, C., & Hunter, M. (2014). The role of resilience in adjustment and coping with chronic pain. *Rehabilitation Psychology, 59*, 360–365.

Pasero, C., & Portenoy, R. K. (2011). Neurophysiology of pain and analgesia and the pathophysiology of neuropathic pain. In C. Pasero & M. McCaffery (Eds.), *Pain assessment and pharmacologic management* (pp. 1–12). St Louis, MO: Mosby/Elsevier.

Phillips, R. L., Short, A., Kenning, A., Dugdale, P., Nugus, P., McGowan, R., & Greenfield, D. (2014). Achieving patient-centered care: The potential and challenge of the patient-as-professional role. *Health Expectations, 18*, 2616–2628.

Qaseem, A., Wilt, T. J., McLean, R. M., Forciea, M., & Clinical Guidelines Committee of the American College of Physicians. (2017). Noninvasive treatments for acute, subacute, and chronic low back pain: A clinical practice guideline from the American College of Physicians. *Annals of Internal Medicine, 166*(7), 514–530.

Starkweather, A. R., & Pair, V. E. (2013). Decoding the role of epigenetics and genomics in pain management. *Pain Management Nursing, 14*, 358–367.

Walker, L. S., Dengler-Crish, C. M., Rippel, S., & Bruehl, S. (2010). Functional abdominal pain in childhood and adolescence increases risk for chronic pain in adulthood. *Pain, 150*, 568–572.

CHAPTER 2

PAIN NEUROPHYSIOLOGY AND PHENOTYPES

Angela Starkweather

Pain takes on many different forms and can change over time. Pain terminology is important for defining the type of pain and informs the range of different treatment strategies that are most effective. Whether the pain originates from a known cause, such as injury, or has no known cause, the patient's description of their pain can provide insight into potential therapeutic modalities. Additionally, phenotyping, or characterizing the pain by its attributes, can help to identify strategies for reducing pain and improving function. In all situations concerning pain, it is important to provide multimodal options and assist the patient in problem-solving their pain—what makes it better, what makes it worse, and how they can strengthen their own coping skills to maximize their function. In this chapter, the pathophysiology of pain is reviewed along with terminology to guide the clinical descriptions used. Types of pain that arise due to injury, disease, and/or infection are then reviewed along with a description of common signs and symptoms.

▌ Neurophysiology of Pain

In the past, pain was thought to originate from a passive system initiated by stimulation or injury of neural tissue (A-delta and C-fibers), which subsequently sends signals to the spinal cord and brain where pain is interpreted and perceived. This is known as the Cartesian model of pain because it was promoted by the philosopher Descartes (1633/2003) hundreds of years ago. The Cartesian model of pain still holds true when we investigate the neurophysiology of nociceptive and neuropathic pain in animal models and in some situations in humans. Nociceptors are high-threshold sensory receptors of the peripheral somatosensory nervous system that are capable of transducing and encoding noxious stimuli (International Association for the Study of Pain, 2017). Pain that arises due to the activation of nociceptors is referred to as nociceptive pain. This term is in contrast to neuropathic pain in which pain is caused by a lesion or disease of the peripheral or central nervous system. Nociceptive pain serves a useful purpose because it helps humans recognize when there is real or potential tissue damage, such as when touching a hot stove, cutting a finger, or with appendicitis. In these instances, there is an identifiable cause of the pain, and once it is removed, we anticipate that the pain will dissipate quickly. Nociceptive pain is studied in animals by administration of noxious stimuli, whereas neuropathic pain can be induced through surgery or traumatic injury. However, often in the work-up of humans, there is no identifiable source of pain and no pathology that could compromise the health or neurologic function. In other words, people have gone through surgeries or procedures and continue to experience pain long after tissue healing has taken place. In these instances, the pain no longer serves a useful purpose and is viewed as a condition or disease in and of itself.

> ▶ **KEY POINT**
>
> Subjective pain descriptors can provide insight into the potential etiology of pain.

> ▶ **KEY POINT**
>
> The neuromatrix theory of pain helps to explain how variability in the experience of pain is affected by the coordination of the brain and spinal cord as well as the individual's genetic make-up.

Human beings are much more complex than what a rodent model can mimic, and clinical observations have led to more advanced theories to explain the mechanisms of pain under various conditions—particularly because it is well known that the degree of injury in humans does not correlate with the level of pain intensity (Balague, Mannion, Pellise, & Cedraschi, 2012; Guermazi et al., 2012; Register et al., 2012). In 1999, Melzack posited the neuromatrix theory of pain in order to understand the independence between tissue injury and the experience of pain. The neuromatrix theory incorporates the role of pain genomics, each individual's genetic make-up, as producing variability in pain perception as well as coordination among the spinal cord and multiple areas of the brain (prefrontal cortex, motor cortex, somatosensory cortex, insular cortex, limbic system, brain stem, and thalamus) that generate pain. Each area of the brain contributes a different dimension to the experience:

▶ Making sense of pain/pain behavior—prefrontal cortex
▶ Where pain is felt in the body—motor and somatosensory cortex
▶ Emotional aspects—limbic and insular systems
▶ Consciousness of pain—brain stem and thalamus

Each of these dimensions has been studied and verified in humans as playing a significant role in how individuals experience and report pain, including the cognitive-behavioral aspects of pain (Atlas & Wager, 2012; Flor, 2012), the somatosensory aspects of pain (Bushnell et al., 1999; Haggard, Iannetti, & Longo, 2013; Lenoir, Huang, Venadermeeren, Hatem, & Mouraux, 2017), and attention to pain (Bantick et al., 2002; Sloan & Hollins, 2017). This lens is consistent with the biopsychosocial model of pain discussed in Chapter 1 and will be expanded upon throughout the remainder of the book.

> ▶ **KEY POINT**
>
> Multimodal options for treatment should be offered along with assistance in problem-solving the patient's pain.

Phenotyping pain can help in understanding the underlying neuropathophysiology especially regarding whether the pain is caused by peripheral, central, or both pathways. For instance, inflammatory joint pain is primarily a peripherally driven condition that occurs through sensitization of nociceptors by inflammatory mediators, such as proinflammatory cytokines. Non-inflammatory muscle pain, as seen in fibromyalgia, is caused by a centralized mechanism that is independent of peripheral afferent input. Current theories of the transition from acute to chronic pain propose that aberrant neurochemical processing of sensory signals in the central nervous system lowers pain thresholds and amplifies normal sensory signals, thereby leading to hypersensitivity and central sensitization. In addition, the normal descending inhibitory pathways involving the rostral ventromedial medulla, nucleus raphe magnus, and dorsolateral posterior tegmentum are not effective in reducing pain signals (Arnold et al., 2016). These alterations lead to the phenotypic characteristics of chronic pain.

> ▶ **KEY POINT**
>
> Modern understanding of the neurophysiology of pain in humans views the brain as the central area that generates pain, with multiple areas providing unique dimensions of the pain experience.

Phenotyping Pain

Pain phenotyping is the method of gathering and categorizing the various characteristics of pain, which can help to provide insight on potential therapeutic targets. Some of the characteristics are gathered during the physical examination such as:

> ▶ **KEY POINT**
>
> Phenotyping pain can help to identify treatment strategies.

- ▶ Location of pain
- ▶ Intensity of pain (worst pain, least pain, average pain, current pain)
- ▶ Frequency of pain
- ▶ Duration of pain
- ▶ Aggravating and alleviating factors
- ▶ Health/social status at the time of onset (stress, trauma, surgery)

However, other aspects can be extremely helpful in guiding which treatments may be most effective, including:

- ▶ Additional information about the pattern of pain throughout a typical day, week, month, and year
- ▶ Identifying whether other symptoms are associated with the pain, such as anxiety, depression, fatigue, sleep disturbance, or cognitive impairment
- ▶ Detecting whether the pain follows a specific distribution neuroanatomically (specific to neuropathic pain)
- ▶ Evaluating the effect of the pain on psychological, social, and physical functioning
- ▶ Examination of the somatosensory changes associated with the pain and endogenous pain-modulatory processes (such as with quantitative sensory testing)
- ▶ Linking the somatosensory descriptors of the pain (Table 2-1)

TABLE 2-1. Common Pain Terms

Allodynia	Pain because of a stimulus that does not usually provoke pain
Dysesthesia	An unpleasant sensation that is either spontaneous or evoked
Hyperalgesia	Increased pain from a stimulus that usually provokes pain
Hyperesthesia	Increased sensitivity to stimulation (both allodynia and hyperalgesia)
Hypoalgesia	Diminished response to a stimulus that is normally painful
Neuropathic pain	Pain caused by a lesion/disease of the somatosensory nervous system (can be classified as central or peripheral)
Nociception	The neural process of encoding noxious stimuli (pain sensation is not necessarily implied)
Nociceptive pain	Pain because of actual or threatened damage to non-neural tissue and to activation of nociceptors
Nociceptor	High-threshold sensory receptor of the peripheral somatosensory nervous system capable of transducing and encoding noxious stimuli
Pain threshold	Minimum intensity of a stimulus that is perceived as painful
Pain tolerance	Maximum intensity of a pain-producing stimulus that a subject is willing to accept in a given situation
Paresthesia	Abnormal sensation that is either spontaneous or evoked
Sensitization	Increased responsiveness of nociceptor neurons to normal input and/or recruitment of a response to normally subthreshold inputs (can be peripheral and/or central)

In addition to these factors, psychosocial characteristics can be very informative such as evaluating mental health history and current status, educational attainment, health habits, and socioeconomic resources (income, healthcare coverage, access to healthcare services).

By evaluating the whole picture of the pain experience, other symptoms such as sleep quality (Fang, Wu, Chen, Teng, & Tsai, 2019), the patterns of distribution (van Hecke et al., 2015), and how it is impacting the individual's life, the clinician can assess a more thorough list of treatment strategies that may be effective (Edwards et al., 2016).

Common Types of Pain

Musculoskeletal pain, including low back pain, affects millions of people and is the most common type of pain reported across the world. However, other types of pain can afflict individuals and are recognized by their unique characteristics. Some of the more common types of pain are described below.

▌ Complex Regional Pain Syndrome

Complex regional pain syndrome (CRPS) type I, which was once referred to as reflex sympathetic dystrophy, usually develops following traumatic injury to an extremity, such as fracture. Type II CRPS, previously referred to as causalgia, can develop after major nerve damage. Although an inciting event is almost always present, CRPS can occur spontaneously. The upper extremity is more often involved compared with the lower extremity, and fracture is the most frequent precipitating event. Signs and symptoms of CRPS are shown in Table 2-2.

▌ Fibromyalgia

Fibromyalgia is a chronic pain condition caused by abnormal pain processing in the central nervous system that results in widespread pain, allodynia (pain because of a stimulus that does not usually provoke pain) and hyperalgesia (increased pain from a

TABLE 2–2. Complex Regional Pain Syndrome Signs and Symptoms

	Symptoms	Signs
Sensory	Reports of hyperalgesia and/or allodynia	Evidence of hyperalgesia (to pinprick) and/or allodynia (to light touch and/or deep somatic pressure and/or joint movement)
	Hypersensitivity to touch or temperature changes	
	Continuous and throbbing or burning pain, usually in the arm, leg, hand, or foot often in part or all of a limb	
Vasomotor	Reports of temperature asymmetry and/or skin color changes and/or skin color asymmetry	Evidence of temperature asymmetry and/or skin color changes and/or asymmetry
	Changes in skin color, ranging from white and mottled to red or blue	
	Changes in skin texture, which may become tender, thin, or shiny in the affected area	
Sudomotor/ Edema	Reports of edema and/or sweating changes and/or sweating asymmetry	Evidence of edema and/or sweating changes and/or sweating asymmetry
	Alternations between sweaty skin and cold skin	
	Edema of the painful area	
Motor/ Trophic	Reports of decreased range of motion and/or motor dysfunction (weakness, tremor, dystonia) and/or trophic changes (hair, nails, and skin)	Evidence of decreased range of motion and/or motor dysfunction (weakness, tremor, dystonia) and/or trophic changes (hair, nails, skin)
	Muscle spasms, tremors, weakness and atrophy of muscles, difficulty coordinating muscle movement	
	Decreased ability to move the affected body part	

stimulus that usually provokes pain). The core symptoms of fibromyalgia, allodynia and hyperalgesia, are caused by neurochemical imbalances in the central nervous system that lead to augmentation of pain perception (centralized) in multiple locations (widespread) (Arnold et al., 2016; Wolfe et al., 2011). The pain is often described as stabbing, shooting, throbbing, and/or twitching with deep muscular aching but may also include numbness, tingling, and burning sensations (Menzies, 2016; Wolfe et al., 2011). Other symptoms of fatigue, sleep disturbances, sensitivity to touch, light and noise, and/or cognitive disturbances significantly influence perceived pain intensity and impairment on physical functioning and quality of life (Menzies, 2016; Theoharides et al., 2015). The Widespread Pain Index (WPI) and Symptom Severity (SS) scale are used together to diagnose fibromyalgia: a WPI of 7 or greater and SS score of 5 or greater; or WPI of 3 to 6 and SS of 9 or greater (Arnold et al., 2016).

Irritable Bowel Syndrome

Intense, recurrent abdominal (visceral) pain is a predominant symptom of irritable bowel syndrome (IBS), a functional gut disorder that typically manifests in the early adult years (Lacy , Chey, & Lembo, 2015; Longstreth et al., 2006). Although women report more severe IBS-related pain, both younger men and women report more severe pain compared to older adult cohorts (Tang, Yang, Liang, et al., 2012; Tang, Yang, Wang & Lin, et al., 2012). Individuals with IBS-related pain report that pain is the most distressing symptom and has the greatest impact on quality of life (Lacy et al., 2015).

Neuropathy

Neuropathy is damage (disease, trauma, infection, vitamin deficiency, or medication) that affects the motor, sensory, and/or autonomic nerves of the peripheral nervous system. Damage to one nerve is referred to as mononeuropathy, whereas multiple nerve involvement is called polyneuropathy. Motor symptoms include weakness, impaired balance, or coordination. Sensory symptoms may include sensitivity to temperature, numbness, tingling, burning, or shooting pain. Autonomic symptoms can include abnormal heart rate or blood pressure, bladder control, and/or sweating.

> ▶ **KEY POINT**
>
> The brain is not a passive recipient of input from the periphery and spinal cord, as once thought, but is interactive in how pain is understood (as a threat or a nuisance), where it is located and travels, the emotions that result, and our attentiveness to it.

Osteoarthritis

The most common form of arthritis occurs with aging as the cartilage between bones of a joint wear down. The most common sites of osteoarthritis affect weight-bearing joints, including the spine, hips, knees, and/or ankles. Bone microfractures, bone spurs (osteophytes), ligament damage, and synovitis can contribute to pain.

Phantom Limb Pain

Sensation that an amputated or missing limb is still attached, which may include pain, itching, or twitching, is phantom limb pain. Risk factors of phantom limb pain include pain in the region prior to amputation/trauma, anxiety, and depression.

Piriformis Syndrome

Piriformis syndrome is a neuromuscular disorder in which the piriformis muscle pinches the sciatic nerve resulting in pain, numbness, and/or tingling in the buttock with possible extension down the leg.

Postherpetic Neuralgia

Herpes zoster (HZ), or shingles, is an infectious disease caused by reactivation of the varicella-zoster virus (VZV), a highly contagious DNA virus (Johnson & Rice, 2014). Following primary infection by human herpesvirus 3, also known as VZV, the virus can lie dormant in cranial nerve ganglia, dorsal root ganglia, and autonomic ganglia of the entire neuraxis for decades (Kennedy, 2016; Kennedy & Cohrs, 2010). When VZV is reactivated, it travels along the sensory ganglion and propagates in the territory of the innervated epidermis, which typically results in a unilateral erythematous maculopapular rash. The dermatome affected by HZ is often described as being itchy, numb, and/or tender, with or without pain. Half of the people affected by HZ have a rash in the thoracic region; other most common sites are in the trigeminal (typically the ophthalmic branch), cervical, and lumbar regions (Haanpää, Rice, & Rowbotham, 2015). Approximately 48 to 72 hours after the rash erupts and progresses to clear vesicles, pustules form, ulcerate, and then scab over. In immunocompromised individuals, the rash can progress to a disseminated infection (Mallick-Searle, Snodgrass, & Brant, 2016). Usually, HZ is a self-limiting disease and over the ensuing 2 to 3 weeks, the scabs fall off, and the pain resolves.

Postoperative Pain

Acute postoperative pain is an expected phenomenon because of tissue manipulation and injury. However, a significant number of patients experience persistent pain after routine invasive procedures or surgery. Multimodal regimens have been found to be effective in reducing persistent postoperative pain, although the specific components vary based on the patient, setting, and surgical procedure (Chou et al., 2016).

Sciatica

Pain radiating down the path of the sciatic nerve, which branches from the lower back and down each leg, is called sciatica. The pain may be described as sharp, shooting, numbness/tingling, or deep aching. It is most often caused by a herniated disk, spinal stenosis, or a bone spur that causes compression of the nerve.

Trigeminal Neuralgia (aka Tic Douloureux)

Trigeminal neuralgia is altered functioning of the trigeminal nerve resulting in episodes of severe, shooting, or jabbing pain from non-noxious stimuli such as touching the face, chewing, speaking, or brushing the teeth. The function of the trigeminal nerve can be altered by thinning or damage to the myelin sheath of the trigeminal nerve; compression of the trigeminal nerve from an artery, vein, tumor, or other tissue; stroke; surgery; or facial trauma.

REFERENCES

Arnold, L. M., Choy, E., Clauw, D. J., Goldenberg, D. L., Harris, R. E., Helfenstein, M. Jr., . . . Wang, G. (2016). Fibromyalgia and chronic pain syndromes: A white paper detailing current challenges in the field. *Clinical Journal of Pain, 32*, 737–746.

Atlas, L. Y., & Wager, T. D. (2012). How expectations shape pain. *Neuroscience Letters, 520*, 140–148.

Balague, F., Mannion, A. F., Pellise, F., & Cedraschi, C. (2012). Non-specific low back pain. *Lancet, 379*, 482–491.

Bantick, S. J., Wise, R. G., Ploghaus, A., Clare, S., Smith, S. M., & Tracey, I. (2002). Imaging how attention modulates pain in humans using functional MRI. *Brain, 125*, 310–319.

Bushnell, M. C., Duncan, G. H., Hofbauer, R. K., Ha, B., Chen, J. I., & Carrier, B. (1999). Pain perception: Is there a role for somatosensory cortex? *Proceedings of the National Academy of Sciences, 96*, 7705–7709.

Chou, R., Gordon, D. B., de Leon-Casasola, O. A., Rosenberg, J. M., Bickler, S., Brennan, T., . . . Wu, C. L. (2016). Management of postoperative pain: A clinical practice guideline from the American Pain Society, the American Society of Regional Anesthesia and Pain Medicine, and the American Society of Anesthesiologists' Committee on Regional Anesthesia, Executive Committee and Administrative Council. *Journal of Pain, 17*, 131–157.

Descartes, R. (1633/2003). *Treatise of man.* Amherst, NY: Prometheus.

Edwards, R. R., Dworkin, R. H., Turk, D. C., Angst, M. S., Dionne, R., Freeman, R., . . . Yarnitsky, D. (2016). Patient phenotyping in clinical trials of chronic pain treatments: IMMPACT recommendations. *Pain, 157*, 1851–1871.

Fang, S. C., Wu, Y. L., Chen, S. C., Teng, H. W., & Tsai, P. S. (2019). Subjective sleep quality as a mediator in the relationship between pain severity and sustained attention performance in patients with fibromyalgia. *Journal of Sleep Research, e12843.*

Flor, H. (2012). New developments in the understanding and management of persistent pain. *Current Opinion in Psychiatry, 25*, 109–113.

Guermazi, A., Niu, J., Hayashi, D., Roemer, F. W., Englund, M., Neogi, T., . . . Felson, D. T. (2012). Prevalence of abnormalities in knees detected by MRI based observational study (Framingham Osteoarthritis Study). *BMJ, 345*, e5339.

Haanpää, M., Rice, A. S. C., & Rowbotham, M. C. (2015). Treating herpes zoster and postherpetic neuralgia. *Pain Clinical Updates, 23*, 1–8.

Haggard, P., Iannetti, G. D., & Longo, M. R. (2013). Spatial sensory organization and body representation in pain perception. *Current Biology, 23*, R164–R176.

International Association for the Study of Pain. (2017, December 14). *Pain terminology.* Retrieved from https://www.iasp-pain.org/Education/Content.aspx?ItemNumber=1698

Johnson, R. W., & Rice, A. S. C. (2014). Postherpetic neuralgia. *New England Journal of Medicine, 371*, 1526–1533.

Kennedy, P. G. E. (2016). Issues in the treatment of neurological conditions caused by reactivation of varicella zoster virus (VZV). *Neurotherapeutics, 13*, 509–513.

Kennedy, P. G. E., & Cohrs, R. J. (2010). Varicella-zoster virus human ganglionic latency—A current summary. *Journal of Neurovirology, 16*, 411–418.

Lacy, B. E., Chey, W. D., & Lembo, A. J. (2015). New and emerging treatment options for irritable bowel syndrome. *Gastroenterology and Hepatology, 11*(4 Suppl. 2), 1–19.

Lenoir, C., Huang, G., Venadermeeren, Y., Hatem, S. M., & Mouraux, A. (2017). Human primary somatosensory cortex is differentially involved in vibrotaction and nociception. *Journal of Neurophysiology, 118*, 317–330.

Longstreth, G. F., Thompson, W. G., Chey, W. D., Houghton, L. A., Mearin, F., & Spiller, R. C. (2006). Functional bowel disorders. *Gastroenterology, 130*(5), 1480–1491.

Mallick-Searle, T., Snodgrass, B., & Brant, J. M. (2016). Postherpetic neuralgia: Epidemiology, pathophysiology, and pain management pharmacology. *Journal of Multidisciplinary Healthcare, 9*, 447–454.

Melzack, R. (1999). From the gate to the neuromatrix. *Pain, S6*, S121–S126.

Menzies, V. (2016). Fibromyalgia syndrome: Current considerations in symptom management. *American Journal of Nursing, 116*, 24–32.

Register, B., Pennock, A. T., Ho, C. P., Strickland, C. D., Lawand, A., & Philoppon, M. J. (2012). Prevalence of abnormal hip findings in asymptomatic participants. *American Journal of Sports Medicine, 40*, 2720–2724.

Sloan, P., & Hollins, M. (2017). Attention and pain: Are auditory distractors special? *Experimental Brain Research, 235*, 1593–1602.

Tang, Y. R., Yang, W. W., Liang, M. L., Xu, X. Y., Wang, M. F., & Lin, L. (2012). Age-related symptom and life quality changes in women with irritable bowel syndrome. *World Journal of Gastroenterology, 18*, 7175–7183.

Tang, Y. R., Yang, W. W., Wang, Y. L., & Lin, L. (2012). Sex differences in the symptoms and psychological factors that influence quality of life in patients with irritable bowel syndrome. *European Journal of Gastroenterology and Hepatology, 24*, 702–707.

Theoharides, T. C., Tsilioni, I., Arbetman, L., Panagiotidou, S., Steward, J. M., Gleason, R. M., & Russell, I. J. (2015). Fibromyalgia syndrome in need of effective treatments. *Journal of Pharmacology and Experimental Therapy, 355*, 255–263.

van Hecke, O., Kamerman, P. R., Attal, N., Baron, R., Bjournsdottir, G., Bennett, D. L., . . . Smith, B. H. (2015). Neuropathic pain phenotyping by international consensus (NeuroPPIC) for genetic studies: A NeuPSIG systematic review, Delphi survey, and expert panel recommendations. *Pain, 156*, 2337–2353.

Wolfe, F., Clauw, D. J., Fitzcharles, M. A., Goldenberg, D. L., Hauser, W., Katz, R. S., . . . Winfield, J. B. (2011). Fibromyalgia criteria and severity scales for clinical and epidemiological studies: A modification of the ACR preliminary diagnostic criteria for fibromyalgia. *Journal of Rheumatology, 38*, 1113–1122.

CHAPTER 3

PAIN ASSESSMENT, CLINICAL HISTORY, AND EXAMINATION

Paula S. McCauley

CASE STUDY You are a novice Advanced Practice Registered Nurse and have been hired by the orthopedic service in your organization to establish a service for pain management. Your first referral is Marie Smith, a 58-year-old female who presented to the emergency department for evaluation of severe low back pain. Her work-up is positive for spinal stenosis and degenerative disk disease at L5-S1. The orthopedist has informed her that she is not a surgical candidate and opted to treat her medically. He prescribed ibuprofen 800 mg 4 times a day and referred her to your pain management service for further evaluation.

As a new provider, where do you start?

Introduction: Pain Assessment

The International Association for the Study of Pain (IASP, 2017) defines pain as a combined sensory, emotional, and cognitive phenomenon: "an unpleasant sensory and emotional experience that we primarily associate with tissue damage or describe in terms of such damage, or both." Pain is a personal, subjective experience influenced by cultural beliefs and other psychological variables (IASP, 2017). Pain is the most common symptom that brings patients to see a provider, and it is often the first sign of an ongoing pathologic process. Depending on the individual circumstances, the same physical lesion or disease state can produce different levels of pain and need for pain relief.

> ▶ **KEY POINT**
>
> You, as the provider they have sought out for care of their circumstances, must keep in mind that the **patient's subjective reporting of pain, not your impression of their pain, is the basis for pain assessment and treatment** (Gomella & Haist, 2007).

Pain medicine has been shaped largely by the biopsychosocial model, first identified by Gordon Waddell in 1987. The biopsychosocial model established that clinicians need to understand pain from the biomedical perspective as well as the impact of the patient's perception and their social context. Pain includes three distinct components: a sensory-discriminatory component, a motivational-affective component, and a cognitive-evaluative component. This framework requires that you have an understanding of the characteristics of the pain, the psychological responses to pain, how and why the pain has changed this person's life, and the implications for recovery (Azari, Zevin, & Potter, 2007).

Pain management has more recently been shaped by patient- and family-centered care. The Agency for Healthcare Research and Quality produced a guide of evidence-based strategies through its Patient and Family Advisory Council that promotes patient- and family-centered care and includes the domain of pain management. Evaluation of the patients' perspective of a need for help with pain-centered care and healthcare providers' focus on pain management revealed major gaps in care. Patients focused on pain assessment, explanation of therapies, and adjunct therapies. Healthcare providers focused on aspects such as medication administration, or reduction in call light usage. Based on their evaluation, the council created a bundle of strategies that may guide development of a personalized plan of care for pain management. These strategies include a redesigned pain management assessment, a menu of pain control, and comfort options (Bookout, Staffileno, & Budzinsky, 2016).

For everyday clinical practice, it is necessary to have outcome measures that are practical and comprehensive enough to be easily used for all patients. Your initial assessment must establish if the pain is acute or chronic and the adverse effects it has created for the patient including physiologic, emotional, and psychological aspects. Your assessment must be systematic, comprehensive, and include evaluation of all the following: (1) type, (2) frequency, (3) location, (4) intensity, (5) modifying factors, (6) effects of treatments, (7) functional impact, and (8) psychosocial impact on the patient. There are multiple instruments available to assess pain. A comprehensive approach to the measurement of pain will include a combination of instruments such as verbal rating scales, numeric rating scales (NRSs), behavioral observation scales, and physiologic responses (Fink, 2000; Gomella & Haist, 2007; Melzack & Katz, 2001; Turk et al., 2003).

One example of a comprehensive approach is based on the Initiative on Methods, Measurement, and Pain Assessment in Clinical Trials (Turk et al., 2003) recommendations. The IMMPACT recommended six core outcome domains: pain, physical functioning, emotional functioning, patient ratings of improvement and satisfaction with treatment, other symptoms and adverse events during treatment, and patient's disposition and characteristics data (Table 3-1; Turk et al., 2003).

Based on the IMMPACT recommendations, the Norwegian Pain Society created a 4-page, 31-item screening questionnaire that covers the IMMPACT-recommended outcome domains. The questionnaire includes questions on coping and catastrophizing, health-related quality of life, economic impact of the pain condition, social security status, and any ongoing litigation or compensation process (Turk et al., 2003).

█ Classification of Pain

█ Acute Pain

Acute pain is caused by noxious stimulation because of injury, a disease process, or the abnormal function of muscle or viscera. The most common forms of acute pain include posttraumatic, postoperative, and obstetric pain as well as pain associated

Table 3-1. The Initiative on Methods, Measurement, and Pain Assessment in Clinical Trials (IMMPACT)-Recommended Six Core Outcome Domains

- *Pain intensity* rated on a 0-10 numeric rating scale and the amount of any rescue analgesics used.
- *Physical functioning* assessed by the Brief Pain Inventory pain interference items.
- *Emotional functioning* assessed by Beck Depression Inventory.
- *Patient ratings of improvement* of the pain condition by the patients' global impression of change scale: patient's report of "minimally improved," moderately important is "much improved," and a substantial change is "very much improved."
- *Other symptoms and any adverse events* are documented by using passive capture of spontaneously reported events and open-ended prompts.
- *Patient's dispositions and characteristics data* assessed in accord with the CONSORT recommendations.

Adapted from Vrooman, B. M, & Rosenquist, R. W. (2013) Chronic pain management. In J. F. Butterworth, D. C. Mackey, & J. D. Wasnick (Eds.), *Morgan & Mikhail's clinical anesthesiology* (6th ed.). New York, NY: McGraw-Hill.

> ▶ **KEY POINT**
>
> The initial assessment when evaluating and classifying pain is to differentiate if it is acute, chronic, or a combination of both. Most pain can be further classified as inflammatory or nociceptive, neuropathic, or idiopathic (Azari et al., 2007).

with acute medical illnesses, such as myocardial infarction, pancreatitis, and renal calculi. Most forms of acute pain are self-limited or resolve with treatment in a few days or weeks (Azari et al., 2007).

Acute pain is typically associated with a systemic neuroendocrine stress response proportional to the pain's intensity. There are two types of acute pain: neuropathic and nociceptive. *Neuropathic pain* arises from disordered nerve signals. It is described by patients as burning, electrical, or shock-like pain. Classic examples are poststroke pain, tumor invasion of the brachial plexus, and herpetic neuralgia. *Nociceptive pain* serves to detect, localize, and limit tissue damage and is further divided into somatic or visceral.

Somatic pain

Somatic pain is the result of direct mechanical or chemical stimulation of nociceptors and normal neural signaling to the brain. It tends to be localized, aching, throbbing, and cramping. The classic example is bone metastases. Deep somatic pain arises from muscles, tendons, joints, or bones and has a dull, aching quality and is less well localized. The intensity and duration of the stimulus affect the degree of localization. Vrooman and Rosenquist (2013) use an example: pain following brief minor trauma to the elbow joint is localized to the elbow, but severe or sustained trauma can cause pain in the whole arm.

Visceral pain

Visceral pain is caused by nociceptors in organ systems such as gastrointestinal and respiratory systems. It may be due to a disease process or abnormal function involving an internal organ or its covering such as parietal pleura, pericardium, or peritoneum. Visceral pain is a deep or colicky type of pain classically associated with disorders or diseases such as pancreatitis or myocardial infarction. It is dull, diffuse, and usually midline, frequently associated with abnormal sympathetic or parasympathetic activity causing symptoms such as nausea, vomiting, sweating, and changes in blood pressure and heart rate (Vrooman & Rosenquist, 2013). Parietal pain is typically sharp and is either localized to the area around the organ or referred to a distant site. Two examples include: pain associated with disease processes involving the peritoneum or pleura over the diaphragm that is frequently referred to the neck and shoulder; or pain from disease processes affecting the parietal surfaces of the peripheral diaphragm that is referred to the chest or upper abdominal wall (Vrooman & Rosenquist, 2013).

On your initial assessment, it is important to document the degree of pain because it identifies patients with severe pain and facilitates treatment. Acute pain assessment will determine duration, location, quality, severity, and exacerbating and relieving factors. Pain assessment should include nonverbal signs, such as tachycardia, tachypnea, and changes in patient expression and movements; the patient's report of pain; and any response to treatment. Periodic pain reassessment is needed because pain is dynamic and changes with time (Ducharme, 2016). Acute pain is typically associated with a systemic neuroendocrine stress response that is proportional to pain intensity. The efferent limb is mediated by the sympathetic nervous and endocrine systems. Sympathetic activation increases sympathetic tone to all viscera and releases catecholamines from the adrenal medulla. Hormonal responses result from increased sympathetic tone and from hypothalamically mediated reflexes. Moderate to severe acute pain may adversely affect perioperative morbidity, mortality, and convalescence (Vrooman & Rosenquist, 2013). Systemic effects can be categorized by systems and are included in Table 3-2.

▍Chronic Pain

Chronic pain persists beyond the usual course of an acute disease or beyond the time normally associated with healing from an acute or subacute injury (usually 2-12 weeks). When pain fails to resolve because of either abnormal healing or inadequate treatment, it becomes *chronic* (Azari et al., 2007). Chronic pain may be nociceptive, neuropathic, or mixed, and psychological mechanisms or environmental factors frequently play a major role. It may be constant, intermittent, or related to physical activity (Vrooman & Rosenquist, 2013). Chronic pain sufferers often experience several types of pain. An illustration of this is chronic low back pain because of osteoarthritis, which is normally classified as inflammatory but may include associated irritation of the nerves and the associated sensory activation in the periphery with sensitization of the central nervous system (Azari et al., 2007). Patients with chronic pain will often have alternations in their neuroendocrine stress responses and have sleep and affective disturbances.

The most common forms of chronic pain include those associated with musculoskeletal disorders; chronic visceral disorders; lesions of peripheral nerves, nerve roots, or dorsal root ganglia (diabetic neuropathy and postherpetic neuralgia); lesions of the central nervous system (stroke, spinal cord injury, and multiple sclerosis); and cancer pain. The pain associated with some disorders such as cancer and chronic back pain is often mixed (Vrooman & Rosenquist, 2013). Systemic responses to chronic pain are included in Table 3-3.

Table 3–2. Systemic Effects of Acute Pain

Cardiovascular effects
Hypertension
Tachycardia
Enhanced myocardial irritability
Increased systemic vascular resistance
Increased cardiac output
Increase in myocardial oxygen demand

Respiratory effects
Increased minute ventilation and work of breathing
Guarding, splinting
Decreased movement of the chest wall = reduced tidal volume and functional residual capacity, atelectasis, intrapulmonary shunting, hypoxemia, and hypoventilation
Reductions in vital capacity = impaired coughing and clearing of secretions

Gastrointestinal and urinary effects
Increased sphincter tone and decreased intestinal and urinary bladder motility
Ileus and urinary retention
Stress ulceration
Nausea, vomiting, and constipation

Endocrine effects
Stress-increased release of catabolic hormones: catecholamines, cortisol, and glucagon
Inhibited release of anabolic hormones (insulin and testosterone)
Negative nitrogen balance, carbohydrate intolerance, increased lipolysis, sodium retention, water retention, and secondary expansion of the extracellular space

Hematologic effects
Increase platelet adhesiveness
Reduced fibrinolysis

Immune effects
Leukocytosis
Stress-related immunodepression may enhance tumor growth and metastasis

Psychological effects
Anxiety and sleep disturbances
Depression
Frustration and anger that may be directed at family, friends, and the medical staff

Adapted from Vrooman, B. M., & Rosenquist, R. W. (2013). Chronic pain management. In J. F. Butterworth, D. C. Mackey, & J. D. Wasnick (Eds.), *Morgan & Mikhail's clinical anesthesiology* (6th ed.). New York, NY: McGraw-Hill.

Table 3–3. Systemic Responses to Chronic Pain

Reduced mobility
Sleep disturbances
Affective disturbances, particularly depression
Decreases or increases in appetite
Psychological stress related to social relationships

Adapted from Vrooman, B. M., & Rosenquist, R. W. (2013). Chronic pain management. In J. F. Butterworth, D. C. Mackey, & J. D. Wasnick (Eds.), *Morgan & Mikhail's clinical anesthesiology* (6th ed.). New York, NY: McGraw-Hill.

CASE STUDY   Back to Ms. Smith, she is brought to the examining room by your medical assistant who had gathered some initial data. Ms. Smith states her pain is lower back, 6/10 at rest, 9/10 with movement, it radiates down into her left hip and buttock. Hervital signs are: temperature 98.5°C; heart rate (HR) 88 beats/min; respiration rate (RR) 18 breaths/min; blood pressure (BP) 146/90. You enter the room to find her standing by the end of the examining table looking pale, tense, and uncomfortable. You introduce yourself and ask if she would like to be seated, she tells you she feels better standing.

Has she given you any clues about her pain, is it acute or chronic?

Have you begun to form your differential for the etiology of her pain?

What pertinent positives and negatives do you need to explore?

You proceed with your pain history.

Pain History

A comprehensive medical history is an important part of the pain history and may reveal important comorbidities that could contribute to a complex pain condition. The level of pain must be assessed to understand what the patient is experiencing and to measure the effectiveness of any treatment. Your history must include questions about onset, quality, duration, and ameliorating or exacerbating factors. The specific pain history must clarify location, intensity, pain descriptors, temporal aspects, and possible pathophysiologic issues (Table 3-4).

Risk factors for various pain syndromes must also be included and may encompass age, fitness level, obesity, occupational exposure, and traumatic events. Comorbid conditions predispose the patient to pain such as inflammatory processes associated with chronic fatigue or fibromyalgia and peripheral neuropathies associated with diabetes or stroke.

Your assessment must incorporate functional limitations. Common functional limitations caused by chronic pain include sleep disturbance, reduced mobility, sexual dysfunction, and decreased ability to perform well in social or work situations. It is important to evaluate work disability caused by pain as you may be asked to provide documentation that may help qualify a patient for

> ▶ **KEY POINT**
>
> It is helpful to begin your history with an open-ended question such as "tell me about your pain." Include additional questions that help the patient tell their story: "what does it feel like, where is it, what words best describe it, what makes it better or worse." Encourage the patient to share his or her story including how the pain impacts their life and function (Fink, 2000).

Table 3-4. Pain Characteristics

- Location: Where is the pain?
- How intense is the pain?
- Description of the pain (e.g., burning, aching, stabbing, shooting, throbbing)
- How did the pain start?
- How long does it last?
- What relieves or reduces the pain?
- What aggravates the pain?

Table 3-5. Functional Assessments

- Sleep. Physical function, ability to work. Finances/economy, mood, family life, social life, sex life.
- What treatments have been received? Effects of treatments? Any adverse effects?
- Depression?
- Worries about the outcome of the pain condition and overall health?
- Any litigation or compensation process?

entitlements that could improve his or her living situation. Advocacy for disability benefits, vocational retraining, and other community services are all part of comprehensive care (National Institutes of Health, 2016).

Examples of functional assessments are included in Table 3-5.

Physical Examination

Your physical examination will provide additional information as you establish your differential diagnosis and begin to formulate your plan (Breivik et al., 2008). As with your history, a comprehensive physical examination is important and must include the following:

1. General physical examination, including vital signs, temperature, and head to toe assessment.
2. Specific pain evaluation using a validated scale with specific and well-defined sensory stimuli for pain thresholds and pain tolerance.
3. A comprehensive neurologic examination, incorporating sensory and motor deficits, and strength. It must include sensory testing; cold allodynia, heat allodynia, mechanical allodynia, hyperalgesia, and temporal summation of pain stimuli.
4. A systematic musculoskeletal system examination: range of motion, inflammation, edema, symmetry, and tenderness.
5. Assessment of psychological factors: depression, anxiety, insomnia, weight gain or loss.

Your physical examination will identify not only the origin of the pain but also the associated systemic impact and impairment (Breivik et al., 2008).

Assessment Instruments

The most common pain assessment instrument asks the patient to rate pain intensity on a numeric scale from 0 to 10 (or 0-100), 0 representing no pain and 10 representing unbearable pain. Pictorial or visual analog scale (VAS) may also be used and are particularly useful for children, adults with low literacy, and elderly patients. Both visual and numeric analog scales have been evaluated, and these scales are helpful for clarifying the relationship between pain and activity, the effectiveness of pain treatments, and the pattern of the patient's pain.

Commonly used instruments include the Brief Pain Inventory (BPI), the Pain Disability Index (PDI), the VAS, and the McGill Pain Inventory (MPQ). The MPQ and VAS are frequently used self-rating instruments for the measurement of pain in clinical and research settings. The MPQ is designed to assess the multidimensional nature of pain experience and is a reliable, valid, and consistent measurement tool. When the time to obtain information from patients is limited and when more information than simply the intensity of pain is desired, the short-form version of MPQ is used. Because of the complexity of these instruments and the time needed to perform, Krebs et al. (2009) derived from the BPI a three-item scale that assesses average Pain, interference with Enjoyment of life, and General activity (PEG). This scale is well suited for more rapid assessments in a primary or ambulatory care setting and provides a foundation upon which chronic pain assessment can begin (Gomella & Haist, 2007; Melzack & Katz, 2001; Turk et al., 2003).

Several tests have been developed to assess functional limitations or impairment, disability, and quality of life. These include the Multidimensional Pain Inventory, Medical Outcomes Survey 36-Item Short Form, PDI, and Oswestry Disability Index (Gomella & Haist, 2007; Melzack & Katz, 2001; Turk et al., 2003).

█ Psychosocial Evaluation

Emotional disorders are commonly associated with chronic pain and often result in varying degrees of psychological distress (Vrooman & Rosenquist, 2013). Screening for mental health disorders and any substance use disorders is imperative. Associated depression and anxiety occur frequently with acute and chronic pain. Determining the contribution of depression to the suffering associated with pain is important. Both the pain and emotional distress need to be treated. Treatment of comorbid mental health problems results in better clinical outcomes in overall pain management (Azari et al., 2007).

> ▶ **KEY POINT**
>
> When pain intensity, characteristics, or duration are disproportionate to disease or injury, or when psychological or social issues or both are apparent, a psychosocial evaluation is necessary.

The most commonly used psychological tests are the Minnesota Multiphasic Personality Inventory (MMPI) and the Beck Depression Inventory. The MMPI can confirm clinical impressions about the role of psychological factors. These evaluations help clarify the role of behavioral factors. There are several validated screening tools for primary care, including the single-question drug and alcohol screeners. The Alcohol Use Disorders Identification Test and the Drug Abuse Screen Test are useful, validated questionnaires and have been shown to be 81% sensitive and 79% specific for the detection of unhealthy alcohol use for the detection of a drug use disorder (Azari et al., 2007).

█ Specific Diagnostic Studies

Additional diagnostic studies will be addressed in upcoming chapters but may include nerve blocks, nerve conduction tests, pharmacologic tests, conventional radiography, computerized tomography, and magnetic resonance imaging.

Pain Assessment in Special Populations

Pediatrics

The first step in the treatment of pain in children is to quantify the severity of symptoms. Infants and young children are especially challenging. Specific pain scales have been developed for children at different developmental stages. Familiarity with and application of these pain scales facilitates treatment of pain and anxiety in children of all ages. Auerbach (2016) provides the following scale for consideration.

The COMFORT pain scale

The COMFORT scale measures distress in unconscious and ventilated infants, children, and adolescents. It incorporates nine indicators: alertness; calmness or agitation; respiratory distress; crying; physical movement; muscle tone; facial tension; arterial pressure; and heart rate. Based on the behaviors exhibited by the patient, each indicator is scored between 1 and 5. The sum of scores can range between 9 and 45, and a score of 17 to 26 generally indicates adequate sedation and pain control.

Face–Legs–Activity–Cry–Consolability

The Face–Legs–Activity–Cry–Consolability tool is a validated tool for scoring postoperative pain in infants and children 2 months to 7 years of age. The instrument incorporates five categories of pain behaviors: facial expression; leg movement; activity; cry; and consolability.

The CRIES Pain Scale

The CRIES Pain Scale is validated for neonates, from 32 weeks of gestational age to 6 months. Each of five categories is scored from 0 to 2: crying; requires O_2 for saturation below 95%; increased vital signs (arterial pressure and heart rate); expression—facial; and sleepless (Auerbach, 2016).

Geriatric Patients

Guidelines published by the American Geriatrics Society recommend that the initial presentation or admission of an older person to any healthcare service should include assessment for evidence of pain (American Geriatrics Society Panel on Persistent Pain in Older Persons, 2002). Persistent pain may affect physical function, psychosocial function, or other aspects of quality of life, and each patient should undergo a comprehensive pain assessment. For patients who are cognitively intact, pain assessments should use direct questioning of the patient. Quantitative assessment of pain should be recorded using a standard pain scale such as a VAS, where a patient can indicate where along the continuum their pain lies.

Cognitive impairment

Cognitive impairment, delirium, dementia, or stroke can present substantial challenges to pain assessment. Commonly available instruments are used in patients with cognitive impairment. Patients with severe cognitive impairment may represent substantial challenges. These individuals often can and do make their needs known in simple yes or no answers or behavioral changes such as grimacing, groaning, or increased agitation. Those with profound aphasia can often provide accurate and reliable answers to yes and no questions. For these patients, it is important to be creative in establishing communication methods for the purpose of pain assessment. Patients should be observed for pain-related behaviors during movement. Unusual behavior in a patient with severe dementia should trigger assessment for pain as a potential cause. In cognitively impaired and nonverbal patients, pain assessment should also include observation or history from caregivers (Kane, Ouslander, Resnick, & Malone, 2013).

The MOBID-2 Pain Scale for the assessment of pain in persons in nursing homes and patients with dementia is a useful behavioral pain assessment tool for older persons with dementia. It is based on patients' behavior in connection with standardized active, guided movements of different body parts and pain behavior related to internal organs, head, and skin (Ferrell, 2017).

Critical Care

Pain is common among patients with critical illness. Despite the wide availability of effective treatments for pain, assessing pain in critically ill patients can be challenging because factors such as delirium, endotracheal tubes, and sedation frequently prevent clear communication about pain (Brummel & Girard, 2017). The 2013 Society of Critical Care Medicine clinical practice guidelines on the management of pain, agitation, and delirium in the ICU suggest that the NRS be used to assess pain when patients are able to self-report. Self-reporting may not be possible among those who are critically ill because of the presence of endotracheal tubes, sedation, or delirium. Several instruments have been developed and validated to aid clinicians in identifying the presence of pain in critically ill patients (Stoltenberg & Joffe, 2016).

The two most widely studied pain assessment tools for use in patients in the ICU are the Behavioral Pain Scale and the Critical Care Pain Observation Tool. Both utilize nonverbal cues and patient behaviors, facial expressions, body movements, and compliance with mechanical ventilation to establish the presence of pain. In situations where the clinician is unsure if a patient is having pain, a trial of an analgesic medication can be used to assess for a decrease in the suspected pain-related behaviors such as tachycardia or tachypnea (Brummel & Girard, 2017).

Palliative/End-of-Life Care

Great emphasis has been placed on addressing dying patients' pain. The frequency of symptoms varies by disease and other associated factors. The most common physical and psychological symptoms among terminally ill patients include pain, fatigue, insomnia, anorexia, dyspnea, depression, anxiety, nausea, and vomiting. In the last days of life, terminal delirium is also common (Lawlor, Lawlor, & Reis-Pina, 2018).

The frequency of pain among terminally ill patients varies significantly. One meta-analysis of adults with advanced or terminal illness found pain prevalence of 30% to 94% in patients with cancer, compared to 21% to 77% for chronic obstructive pulmonary disease, 14% to 78% for congestive heart failure, 11% to 83% for end-stage renal disease, 14% to 63% for dementia, and 30% to 98% for acquired immunodeficiency syndrome (van den Beuken-van Everdingen, Hochstenbach, Joosten, Tjan-Heijinen, & Janssen, 2016).

Uncontrolled pain has been reported by patients seen both in the outpatient cancer center and in hospitalized patients with cancer. In patients with cancer, pain may be the only symptom present prior to diagnosis and can also indicate the recurrence or spread of the disease. Pain was the most common symptom among patients with cancer referred to a palliative care service.

As many as 30% to 50% of patients receiving active anticancer therapy experience pain. Pain resulting from the tumor burden occurs in approximately 65% to 85% of patients with advanced cancer. Pain mechanism, incidental occurrences, psychological distress, addictive behavior, and cognitive dysfunction have been indicated as factors associated with higher ratings of pain intensity (Knudsen et al., 2009). There is no universally accepted assessment tool for cancer pain but the revised Edmonton Classification System for Cancer Pain characterizing these factors can be used to guide pain management (Lawlor, et al., 2018).

Family and caregivers

Although pain is an individual experience, family and caregiver contribution in the assessment of pain may be helpful. Family and caregivers are an excellent source of qualitative information about general behavior, medication usage, and actions that seem to aggravate or reduce pain, especially among those patients unable to communicate their pain experience. Among patients with cognitive impairment, the history is often only obtainable from family or close caregivers.

CASE STUDY Now let's review what we have learned from Ms. Smith. Her pain has been persistent for 2 years. She had no trauma or injury that precipitated the onset. Her usual level is 6/10 but flares to 9/10 with movement, it radiates down her leg. The pain is worse when sitting or lying down, with bending and lifting, it is a bit better when standing, although she develops spasms when she stands and walks for long periods of time. The ibuprofen does not help and recently she has developed gastrointestinal distress because of it. She has tried oxycodone on several occasions with minimal effect but would rather not take it because she doesn't like feeling high. She has not been able to work for the past 6 months, does no regular physical activity, and often sleeps in the recliner because of it. She is married but has had no sexual relations for the past year and her marriage has become strained by the chronic pain. She is anxious and feels depressed as it has impacted all aspects of her life.

Have you formed a differential?

What diagnostics would you consider?

What comprehensive plan will you develop with her?

As we move on to the next chapters, we will explore additional options.

▌Conclusion

The patient's subjective reporting of pain, not the clinician's impression of their pain, is the basis for pain assessment and treatment. Clinicians need to approach pain from the biomedical perspective with its three distinct components: a sensory-discriminatory component, a motivational-affective component, and a cognitive-evaluative component. The use of evidence-based strategies that promote patient- and family-centered care and include the domains of pain management will result in comprehensive pain assessment and set the stage for successful management strategies. Developing goals of care with the patient will be very important in that success.

REFERENCES

American Geriatrics Society Panel on Persistent Pain in Older Persons. (2002). The management of persistent pain in older persons. *Journal of American Geriatrics Society, 50,* S205–S224.

Auerbach, P. S. (2016). Pain management and procedural sedation in infants and children. In J. E. Tintinalli, J. Stapczynski, O. Ma, D. M. Yealy, G. D. Meckler, & D. M. Cline (Eds.), *Tintinalli's emergency medicine: A comprehensive study guide* (8th ed.). New York, NY: McGraw-Hill.

Azari, S., Zevin, B., & Potter, M. B. (2007). Chronic pain management in vulnerable populations. In T. E. King & M. B. Wheeler (Eds.), *Medical management of vulnerable and underserved patients: Principles, practice, and populations* (2nd ed.). New York, NY: McGraw-Hill.

Bookout, M. L., Staffileno, B. A., & Budzinsky, C. M. (2016). Partnering with a patient and family advisory council to improve patient care experiences with pain management. *Journal of Nursing Administration, 46*(4), 181–186.

Breivik, H., Borchgrevink, P. C., Allen, S. M., Rosseland, L. A., Romundstad, L., Breivik Hals, E. K., . . . Stubhaug, A. (2008). Assessment of pain. *BJA: British Journal of Anaesthesia, 101*(1), 17–24. doi:10.1093/bja/aen103

Brummel, N. E., & Girard, T. D. (2017). Critical care. In: J. B. Halter, J. G. Ouslander, S. Studenski, K. P. High, S. Asthana, M. A. Supiano, & C. Ritchie (Eds.), *Hazzard's geriatric medicine and gerontology* (7th ed.). New York, NY: McGraw-Hill.

Ducharme, J. (2016) Acute pain management. In J. E. Tintinalli, J. Stapczynski, O. Ma, D. M. Yealy, G. D. Meckler, & D. M. Cline (Eds.), *Tintinalli's emergency medicine: A comprehensive study guide* (8th ed.). New York, NY: McGraw-Hill.

Ferrell, B. A. (2017). Pain management. In: J. B. Halter, J. G. Ouslander, S. Studenski, K. P. High, S. Asthana, M. A. Supiano, & C. Ritchie (Eds.), *Hazzard's geriatric medicine and gerontology* (7th ed.). New York, NY: McGraw-Hill.

Fink, R. (2000). Pain assessment: The cornerstone to optimal pain management. *Proceedings (Baylor University Medical Center), 13*(3), 236–239.

Gomella, L. G., & Haist, S. A. (Eds.). (2007). *Clinician's pocket reference: The Scut Monkey* (11th ed.). New York, NY: McGraw-Hill.

International Association for the Study of Pain. (2017). *IASP terminology*. Retrieved from http://www.iasp-pain.org/terminology?navItemNumber=576#Pain

Kane, R. L., Ouslander, J. G., Resnick, B., & Malone, M. L. (Eds.). (2013). *Essentials of clinical geriatrics* (8th ed.). New York, NY: McGraw-Hill.

Knudsen, A. K., Aass, N., Fainsinger, R., Caraceni, A., Klepstad, P., Jorddhoy, M., . . . Kaasa, S. (2009). Classification of pain in cancer patients—A systematic literature review. *Palliative Medicine, 23*(4), 295–308.

Krebs, E. E., Lorenz, K. A., Bair, M. J., Damush, T. M., Wu, J., Sutherland, J. M., . . . Kroenke, K. (2009). Development and initial validation of the PEG, a three-item scale assessing pain intensity and interference. *Journal of General Internal Medicine, 24*(6), 733–738. doi:10.1007/s11606-009-0981-1

Lawlor, P. G., Lawlor, N. A., & Reis-Pina, P. (2018). The Edmonton classification system for cancer pain: A tool with potential for an evolving role in cancer pain assessment and management. *Expert Review of Quality of Life in Cancer Care, 3*(2–3), 47–64. doi:10.1080/238 09000.2018.1467211

Melzack, R., & Katz, J. (2001). The McGill pain questionnaire: Appraisal and current status. In D. C. Turk & R. Melzack (Eds.), *Handbook of pain assessment* (pp. 35–52). New York, NY: Guilford Press.

National Institutes of Health. (2016). National pain strategy, a comprehensive population health-level strategy for pain. Washington, DC: Department of Health and Human Services. Retrieved from https://painconsortium.nih.gov/

Stoltenberg, E., & Joffe, A. (2016). Analgesia, sedation, and neuromuscular blockade. In: J. M. Oropello, S. M. Pastores, & V. Kvetan (Eds.), *Critical care.* New York, NY: McGraw-Hill.

Turk, D. C., Dworkin, R. H., Allen, R. R., Bellamy, N., Brandenburg, N., Carr, D. B., . . . Witter, J. (2003) Core outcome domains for chronic pain clinical trials: IMMPACT recommendations. *Pain, 106,* 337–345.

van den Beuken-van Everdingen, M. H., Hochstenbach, L. M., Joosten, E. A., Tjan-Heijinen, V. C., & Janssen, D. J. (2016). Update on prevalence of pain in patients with cancer: Systematic review and meta-analysis. *Journal of Pain and Symptom Management, 51*(6), 1070–1090.

Vrooman, B. M., & Rosenquist, R. W. (2013). Chronic pain management. In J. F Butterworth, D. C. Mackey, & J. D. Wasnick (Eds.), *Morgan & Mikhail's clinical anesthesiology* (6th ed.). New York, NY: McGraw-Hill.

CHAPTER 4

DIAGNOSTIC TESTING AND IMAGING OF PAIN

Charan Singh and Edward Gillis

Introduction

In the United States, chronic pain affects more than 100 million adults and accounts for approximately $600 billion annually in medical costs and lost productivity (Martucci & Mackey, 2017). Lower back pain is extremely prevalent, with a mean prevalence of 31% for individuals worldwide and a lifetime prevalence between 11% and 84% (Hoy et al., 2012).

In the United States, approximately 80% will be affected at some point in their lives with chronic lower back pain, accounting for 12% to 15% of healthcare visits (Hoy et al., 2012). Imaging has allowed for increased understanding and management of chronic pain, particularly lower back pain. Diagnostic imaging is used to identify the source of pain and/or pathology that could compromise neurologic functioning. Common imaging studies include:

- ▶ Plain radiographs
- ▶ CT/CT myelogram
- ▶ CT/MR diskography
- ▶ Bone scan/positron emission tomography (PET)
- ▶ MRI

Common indications of imaging studies in chronic pain:

- ▶ Low back and joint pain
- ▶ Osteoarthritis
- ▶ Malignancy
- ▶ Sequela of trauma
- ▶ Neuropathy/myelopathy
- ▶ Image-guided interventions such as epidural steroid injections, vertebroplasty/kyphoplasty.

Chronic spine pain is generally secondary to degenerative changes, with osteophyte formation, disk and facet degeneration resulting in narrowing of the central canal and impingement on exiting nerve roots.

Plain Radiographs/CT

The imaging of uncomplicated chronic pain generally begins with radiographs (Figure 4-1). Presence of osteophytes, spondylolisthesis, dynamic instability, and disk space reduction usually correlates with underlying spinal/neural foramina stenosis. The oblique "Scottie dog" views (Figure 4-2) help determine spondylolysis (pars defects), facet arthropathy, and neural foramina compromise. If there is concern for fracture, superior bony anatomy can be achieved with a noncontrast CT examination.

Magnetic Resonance Imaging

MRI is widely used as a standard method for evaluating spine abnormalities and disease. MRI is ordered with contrast (gadolinium) to improve the clarity of soft tissue images, particularly inflammation, tumors, blood vessels, and, for some organs, blood supply. In general, the decision to include contrast is based on the differential diagnosis and medical condition of the patient, with recommendations provided in Table 4-1.

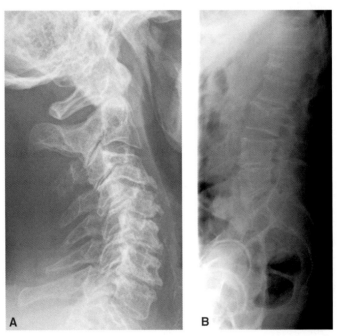

Figure 4-1. Lateral views of (A) the cervical and (B) lumbar spine in neutral position. Cervical spine with severe degenerative spondylosis. Lumbar spine with severe degenerative spondylosis, which results in 2 mm retrolisthesis of L2 on L3. Note the chronic compression fracture of L1.

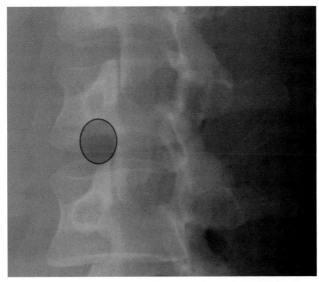

Figure 4-2. Right lateral oblique view of the lumbar spine shows the normal appearance of the "Scottie dog." The transverse process of L3 represents the nose. The pedicle of L3 forms the eye. The inferior L3 articular facet forms the front leg. The superior articular facet of L3 forms the ear. The pars interarticularis, the lamina between the facets, is the neck. Any abnormality at the neck could represent a pars fracture. The circle represents the approximate location of the neural foramen.

Table 4-1. MRI Contrast versus No Contrast

Body Region	Reason for Imaging	MRI with or without Contrast
Brain	Headache/migraine Mental status change/memory loss Seizures, stroke, transient ischemic attack, trauma	MRI brain without contrast
Brain	Cranial nerve lesion Infection Metastatic disease Multiple sclerosis Neurofibromatosis Pituitary involvement	MRI brain with and without contrast
Spine—cervical, thoracic, and/or lumbar	Neck/back pain Disk herniation/radiculopathy Extremity pain/weakness Compression fracture Stenosis Trauma	MRI spine (region) without contrast
Spine—cervical, thoracic, and/or lumbar	Diskitis Mass/lesion Osteomyelitis Postsurgery	MRI spine (region) with and without contrast

(continued)

Table 4-1. MRI Contrast versus No Contrast (*continued*)

Body Region	Reason for Imaging	MRI with or without Contrast
Extremity—nonjoint	Fracture/stress fracture Muscle/tendon tear	MRI (extremity) without contrast
Extremity—nonjoint	Abscess Cellulitis Morton's neuroma Osteomyelitis Soft tissue tumor/mass/ulcer	MRI (extremity) with and without contrast
Extremity—joint	Arthritis Cartilage tear Fracture/stress fracture Internal derangement Joint pain Ligament/meniscal/muscle or tendon tear	MRI (joint) without contrast
Extremity—joint	Abscess Cellulitis Osteomyelitis Tumor/mass/ulcer	MRI (joint) with and without contrast
Pelvis	Pelvic pain Muscle/tendon tear Sacroiliac joints Pelvic pain Adenomyosis/endometriomas Uterine anomalies	MRI pelvis without contrast
Pelvis	Abscess/ulcer Osteomyelitis Adnexal mass Endometrial/ovarian cancer Known fibroids/ovarian cysts	MRI pelvis with and without contrast
Abdomen	Pancreas, gallbladder, liver, ducts	Magnetic resonance cholangiopancreatography without contrast
Abdomen	Kidneys, liver Mass/infection	MRI abdomen with and without contrast
Brachial plexus	Brachial plexus neuropathy	MRI chest without contrast

For the patient with spinal pain, MRI without contrast is indicated in presurgical planning if the patient fails conservative management. If there is a contraindication to MRI, a CT myelogram (Table 4-2) may be obtained. MRI with contrast is indicated in postsurgical patients with ongoing pain/radiculopathy to differentiate residual disk pathology versus scarring.

Table 4-2. Commonly Affected Nerve Roots and Associated Sensorimotor Deficits

Nerve Root	Pain/Numbness	Motor Weakness
C5	Lateral upper arm	Elbow flexion
C6	Lateral forearm and 1st–2nd fingers	Wrist extension
C7	Palm and 3rd finger	Elbow extension
C8	Medial forearm and 4th–5th fingers	Finger flexion
L2	Anterior and medial thigh	Hip flexion and adduction
L3	Anterior thigh and knee	Knee extension and hip flexion and adduction
L4	Anterior and medial calf	Hip extension, flexion, adduction
L5	Lateral leg and medial foot (arch)	Foot dorsiflexion and toe flexion and extension
S1	Posterior thigh and calf, heel and lateral foot	Foot plantarflexion and toe and knee flexion

The MRI protocol for evaluation of the spine in patients with radiculopathy is simple and consists of:

▶ T1 axial and sagittal
▶ T2 axial and sagittal
▶ Sagittal short TI-inversion recovery (STIR)
▶ +/− T1 fat suppression (FS) axial and sagittal if using contrast for evaluation of scar tissue or neoplasm

▌ MRI versus Clinical Findings

The presence of neural foramen narrowing and location of displaced disk are more important in determining the clinical symptoms, whereas the size and extent of the disk correlate poorly with clinical examination. The paramedial disk displacements with neural foramina compromise generally correlate well with the dermatomal distribution of pain (Figure 4-3; Iannuccilli, Prince, & Soares, 2013).

Routine MRI of a normal lumbar intervertebral disk space is shown in Figure 4-4. On T2-weighted sequences, the central disk material (nucleus pulposus) demonstrates

> ▶ **KEY POINT**
>
> It is interesting to know that *nerve compression on an MRI does not necessarily correlate with nerve deficits in all patients, but when deficits are present, they correlate well with the presence of nerve compression on the MRI* (Van de Kelft & van Vyve, 1994).

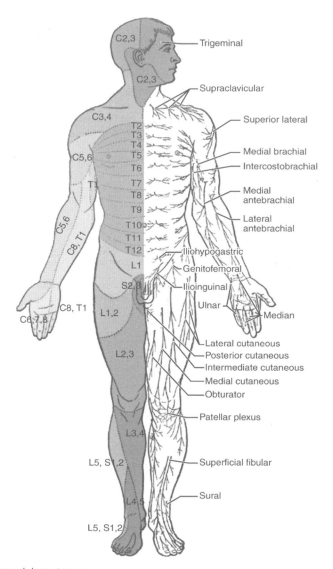

Figure 4-3. Normal dermatomes.

high signal intensity and is surrounded by a peripheral rim of low signal intensity representing the annulus fibrosus.

Common imaging findings of degenerate disk disease with MRI:

- ▶ Facet joint arthropathy (enlarged facet joints because of degenerative arthritis owing to prior trauma or chronic wear and tear)
- ▶ Ligamentum flavum hypertrophy
- ▶ Large osteophytes

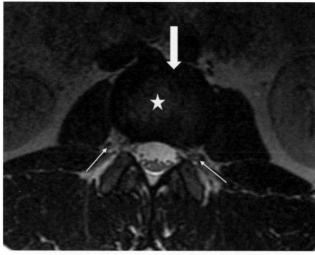

Figure 4-4. Axial T2-weighted image of a normal lumbar intervertebral disk: High signal intensity nucleus pulposus (white star) surrounded by a peripheral low signal intensity annulus fibrosis (thick white arrow) and exiting nerve roots (thin white arrows).

▶ Uncovertebral joint hypertrophy (cervical vertebrae C2-C6 only; enlarged, arthritic uncovertebral joints because of trauma or chronic wear and tear)
▶ Disk herniations and bulges
▶ Posterior and anterior longitudinal ligament calcification and/or hypertrophy
▶ Spondylolysis/listhesis
▶ Neural foraminal compromise

A disk bulge is the result of tears in the annulus with stretching of disk tissue without focal pulposus herniation. Disk bulges can be broad (diffuse) or asymmetric (Figure 4-5).

Disk herniations (Figure 4-6) are the result of trauma, arthritis, and numerous other causes of degenerative lumbar spinal pathology, which can result in compression of the spinal cord and traversing nerve roots to cause varying degrees of pain and discomfort.

Like the lumbar spine, cervical spine degenerative disorder is associated with stenosis of the spinal canal and is frequently seen in the elderly (Janardhana, Rajagopal, & Kamath, 2010; Kang et al., 2011). It consists of similar factors that result in stenosis of the lumbar spine, such as herniated or bulging disks, osteophyte formation, and articular facet arthropathy. Uncovertebral joints are unique to the cervical spine and add an additional element for potential degenerative changes, which result in narrowing of the spinal canal. First, we will look at the normal appearance of the cervical spinal canal (Figure 4-7).

> ▶ **KEY POINT**
>
> The epidural space is the smallest in the upper cervical spine, approximately 1 to 2 mm. Having the patient flex the neck helps widen the posterior epidural space. Correct placement in the epidural space will be denoted by a thin line of contrast along the pedicles or around the nerve root (Figure 4-15).

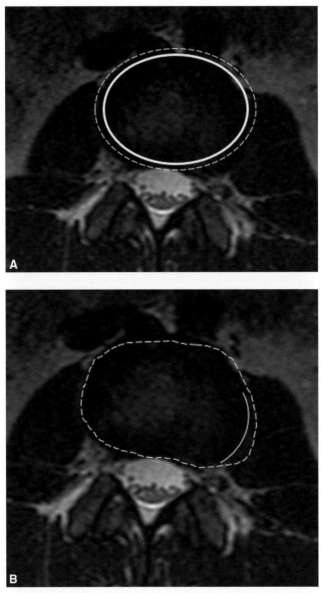

Figure 4-5. Disk bulge: Broad (A)—solid white circle represents the normal disk space and dashed circle represents disk tissue; asymmetric (B)—dashed circle represents disk material with an asymmetric bulge on left and solid curved line represents the margin of the normal disk space.

> ▶ **KEY POINT**
>
> MRI provides superior evaluation of spinal cord abnormalities. Cerebrospinal fluid (CSF) should normally flow freely around the cord. The degree of CSF effacement correlates with the severity of central spinal canal stenosis (Figure 4-9).

One thing to be mindful of, especially when doing transforaminal injections for pain in the cervical spine, is the proximity of the vertebral arteries to the neural foramen. They run in the foramen transversarium, which is located slightly anterolateral to the foramen as seen in Figure 4-8.

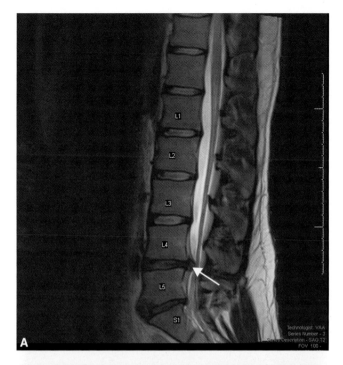

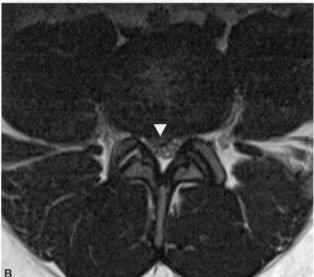

Figure 4-6. MRI sagittal and axial T2-weighted images of the lumbar spine at the L4-L5 level. (A) L4-L5 right paracentral disk protrusion (arrow) resulting in moderate central canal stenosis and (B) impinging on the exiting right L4 nerve root (arrowhead).

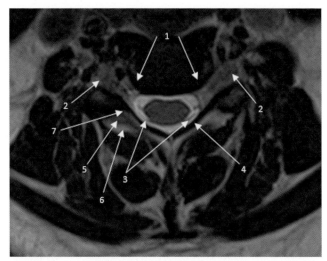

Figure 4-7. Normal cervical spine at the C5 level. 1, Uncovertebral joints; 2, dorsal root ganglion; 3, ligamentum flavum; 4, articular facet joint; 5, superior articular process; 6, inferior articular process; 7, vertebral artery.

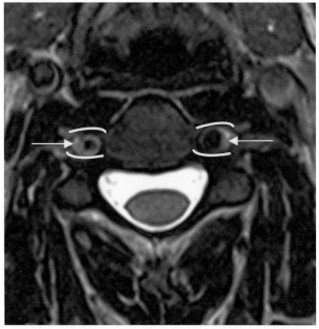

Figure 4-8. Axial T2-weighted image of the cervical spine at the C3-C4 level. The vertebral arteries appear as flow voids on T2-weighted sequences (arrows) located in the foramen transversarium (solid curved lines).

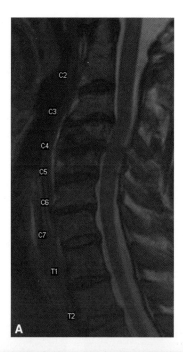

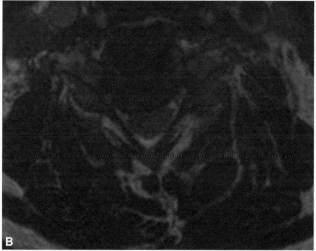

Figure 4-9. A, Sagittal T2-weighted image at midline of the cervical spine (left) and axial T2-weighted image at C4-C5. Severe degenerative spondylosis results in multilevel disk protrusions as seen on sagittal image. B, Axial image shows severe central canal stenosis with uncovertebral joint hypertrophy on the right as well as right paracentral disk protrusion impinging on the exiting nerve root.

▌ Diskography (Provocative Diskography)

Diskogenic pain has been identified in 26% to 39% of patients with low back pain (Anderson & Flanagan, 2000). Lumbar diskography remains a controversial diagnostic technique, but has been concluded to be the most reliable test in diagnosing diskogenic pain (Coppes, Marani, & Thomeer, 1997). It is defined as a procedure in which contrast media are injected into the disk to delineate its morphology and identify if there is an exact and/or similar reproduction of patient's pain.

> ▶ **KEY POINT**
>
> Although normal MRI is the standard for evaluation of spinal cord abnormalities, CT diskography can be used to identify pure foraminal disk herniations and diskogenic pain, and can identify the precise spinal level the pain is originating from.

CT diskography can be useful for the evaluation of painful disk among multiple degenerative disks and helps in surgical planning prior to lumbar fusion or microdiskectomy procedures (Hamasaki et al., 2005). CT diskography is also useful to localize radicular symptoms in presurgical planning (Figure 4-10).

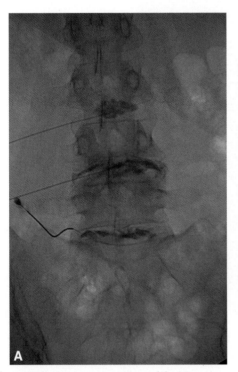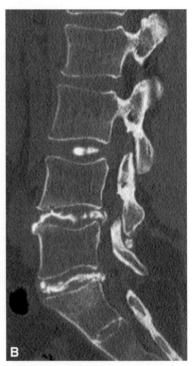

Figure 4-10. Fluoroscopic guidance (A) of Omnipaque contrast injection into the L3-L4, L4-L5, and L5-S1 levels under varying degrees of pressure to correlate radicular pain to specific lumbar levels in presurgical planning. CT diskogram (B) shows normal L3-L4 disk morphology, partial thickness L4-L5 annular tear and full thickness L5-S1 annular tear.

Figure 4-11. Sagittal fused positron emission tomography/computed tomography image in a patient with lower extremity radiculopathy. High fluorodeoxyglucose avidity is present in the lumbar spine at L2 and L3, consistent with metastatic disease in this patient with known prostate cancer.

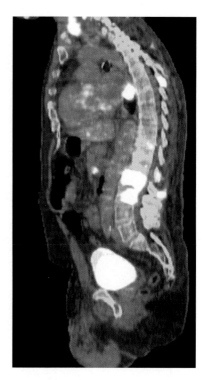

Bone Scan/PET CT Scan

A PET scan uses a small amount of a radioactive drug, or tracer, to show differences between healthy and diseased tissue. One of the most frequently used tracer is known as fluorodeoxyglucose (FDG). A FDG-PET/CT is useful to determine benign from malignant compression fractures and/or assessing for tumor burden (Figure 4-11). If malignancy is suspected, a ^{99m}Tc whole-body bone scan is useful, particularly if one is searching for widespread tumor burden (Figure 4-12).

Imaging Anatomy for Interventions

Imaging with fluoroscopy or CT enables safe and accurate administration of steroid medication in the epidural space either with intralaminar or transforaminal approach as illustrated in Figures 4-13 and 4-14. Similar fluoroscopy guidance is essential in procedures such as vertebroplasty/kyphoplasty, facet injection and ablations, sacroiliac joint injections, and various nerve blocks for pain management (Figure 4-15).

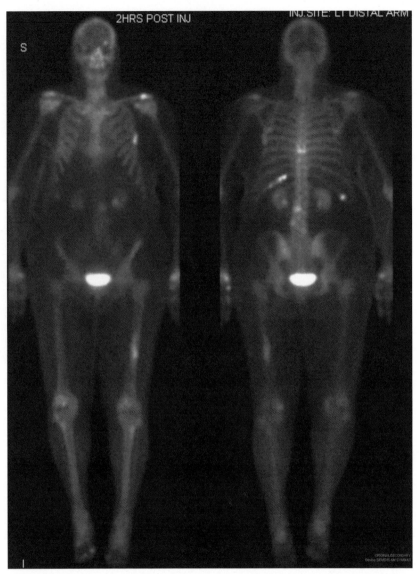

Figure 4-12. ^{99m}Tc whole-body bone scan in a patient with breast cancer with back and thigh pain anterior view (left) and posterior view (right). Increased uptake is seen in the T9 vertebral body, left femur, supraorbital aspect of the skull on the left, left 6th rib, and bilateral 11th ribs. Femoral lesion was found negative for cancer at pathology.

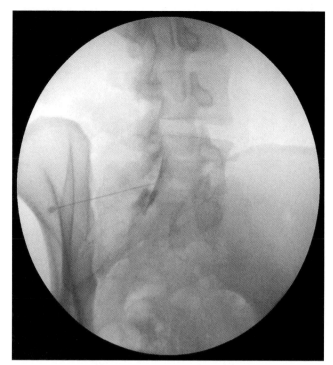

Figure 4-13. Epidural steroid injection. Note the contrast appropriately layering in the epidural space, confirming correct needle location prior to steroid injection.

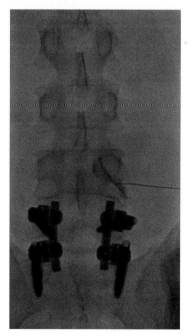

Figure 4-14. Transforaminal injection. Contrast in the right neural foramen confirms correct placement of the needle prior to steroid injection.

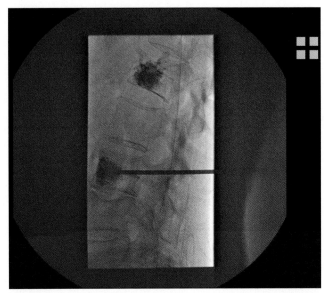

Figure 4-15. Vertebroplasty. Imaging landmarks and anatomy help instillation of cement into fractured vertebrae for pain relief.

▌Conclusion

Imaging plays an important role in the diagnosis, evaluation, and treatment of pain in individuals across age groups. Diagnostic imaging is critical for identifying pathology and potential sources of pain as well as structural instability of the spine. Imaging is used for surgical planning and is critical for interventional pain management techniques to ensure safe and accurate administration of medications or tissue/bone manipulation.

REFERENCES

Anderson, S. R., & Flanagan, B. (2000). Discography. *Current Revision of Pain, 4*, 343–352.

Coppes, M. H., Marani, E., & Thomeer, R. T. W. M. (1997). Innervation of painful lumbar disc. *Spine, 232*, 2342–2350.

Hamasaki, T., Baba, I., Tanaka, S., Sumida, T., Manabe, H., Tanaka, N., & Ochi, M. (2005). Clinical characterizations and radiologic findings of pure foraminal-type cervical disc herniation: CT discography as a useful adjuvant in its precise diagnosis. *Spine, 30*, E591–E596.

Hoy, D., Bain, C., Williams, G., March, L., Brooks, P., Blyth, F., . . . Buchbinder, R. (2012). A systematic review of the global prevalence of low back pain. *Arthritis Rheum, 64*, 2028–2037.

Iannuccilli, J. D., Prince, E. A., & Soares, G. M. (2013). Interventional spine procedures for management of chronic low back pain—A primer. *Seminars in Interventional Radiology, 30*(3), 307–317.

Janardhana, A. P., Rajagopal, R. S., & Kamath, A. (2010). Correlation between clinical features and magnetic resonance imaging findings in lumbar disc prolapse. *Indian Journal of Orthopaedics, 44*(3), 263–269.

Kang, Y., Lee, J. W., Koh, Y. H., Hur, S., Kim, S. J., Chai, J. W., & Kang, H. S. (2011). New MRI grading system for the cervical canal stenosis. *American Journal of Roentgenology, 197*(1), W134–W140.

Martucci, K. T., & Mackey, S. C. (2017). Imaging pain. *Anesthesiology Clinical, 34*(2), 255–269.

Van de Kelft, E., & van Vyve, M. (1994). Diagnostic imaging algorithm for cervical soft disc herniation. *Journal of Neurology, Neurosurgery & Psychiatry, 67*, 724–728.

CHAPTER 5

MULTIMODAL PAIN MANAGEMENT

Kyounghae Kim

The International Association for the Study of Pain (1994) defines pain as "an unpleasant sensory and emotional experience associated with actual or potential tissue damage, or described in terms of such damage." The definition represents that pain does not necessarily mean there is injury and implies the multidimensional nature of pain. Traditionally, management strategies for pain have predominantly focused on pharmacologic and interventional approaches. As pain research is evolving, there is a much greater emphasis on the biobehavioral approach targeting the behavioral/psychological aspects of pain in addition to analgesic medications (Department of Health and Human Services, 2016; Institute of Medicine, 2011). This approach is based on the biopsychosocial model of pain, which is now generally considered the most heuristic perspective on chronic pain (Gatchel, Peng, Peters, Fuchs, & Turk, 2007). As discussed in Chapter 1, the biopsychosocial model concentrates both health and illness, illness being considered the complex interactions of biologic, psychological, and social components (Gatchel, 2005). In brief, the *bio* portion of the model explains the physiology and neurobiology of the nociception and psychosocial components, which include both emotion and cognition (Gatchel et al., 2007). Emotion is the quicker response to nociceptive pain, which is midbrain based, whereas cognition is connected to the emotional experience and may then prompt additional emotional responses and thus magnify the pain experience, thereby perpetuating a vicious cycle of nociceptive stimulus, pain, and functional limitations (Gatchel et al., 2007). The multidimensional nature of chronic pain suggests that a logical management approach is multimodal, which is an integrated multidisciplinary treatment with closely coordinated somatic and psychotherapeutic components (Muller-Schwefe et al., 2017). This chapter provides an overview of the current research evidence on multimodal pain management in the context of perioperative pain, neck pain, chronic low back pain, fibromyalgia, and cancer pain. The reviewed evidence predominantly focuses on the findings from the meta-analyses of randomized controlled trials (RCTs) among adults aged 18 and older with pain conditions. Articles focusing on children and perinatal care were excluded.

> ▶ **KEY POINT**
>
> Multimodal pain management provides the potential for a decrease in pain, opioid consumption, and opioid-related adverse effects by targeting biologic, psychological, and social factors associated with the pain mechanism.

Perioperative Pain

Figure 5-1 depicts the complementary mechanisms of action along the nociceptive pathway by which interventions exert their action to alleviate pain (Manworren, 2015). Multimodal analgesia may offer additive or synergistic effects on greater pain relief and less adverse effects found with analgesics than would a monomodal approach by combining a variety of analgesics and techniques, along with nonpharmacologic

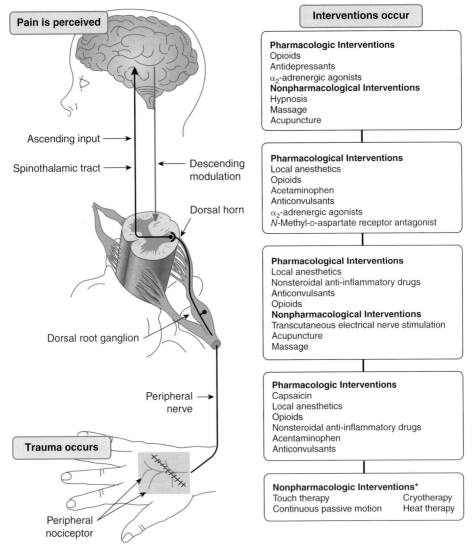

Figure 5-1. The effect of pain management interventions along the nociceptive pain pathway. Adapted with permission from Manworren, R. C. (2015). Multimodal pain management and the future of a personalized medicine approach to pain. *AORN Journal, 101*(3), 311. doi:10.1016/j.aorn.2014.12.009. Copyright ©2015, John Wiley and Sons.

approaches (Chou et al., 2016; Manworren, 2015). Traditional pharmacologic agents include local anesthetics, acetaminophen, and nonsteroidal anti-inflammatory drugs (NSAIDs) including cyclooxygenase-2 inhibitors and opioid analgesics. Nontraditional agents include anticonvulsants, N-methyl-D-aspartate receptor antagonists, α_2-adrenergic agonists, and antidepressants. Per practice guidelines, the choice of medicine, dose, and duration of the treatment should be personalized, yet patients should receive around-the-clock regimens (Chou et al., 2016). Detailed information is provided in Chapter 7. Nonpharmacologic interventions, which are discussed in Chapter 8, generally include transcutaneous electrical nerve stimulation; cognitive behavioral therapy including relaxation methods, guided imagery, and hypnosis; and complementary approaches including acupuncture, massage, and music therapy.

When NSAIDs are used as an adjunct to opioid therapy for perioperative pain, patients tend to have a greater pain reduction compared to the use of either NSAIDs or opioids alone. For example, meta-analysis of 13 RCTs ($n = 782$) supported the finding that single-dose perioperative, intravenous, or intramuscular ketorolac (30- or 60-mg dosage) is an effective adjunct to multimodal analgesia to relieve postoperative pain and reduce opioid consumption (De Oliveira, Agarwal, & Benzon, 2012). The combined regimen reduced immediate postoperative pain with a moderate weighted mean difference (WMD) of -0.64 (95% confidence interval [CI]: -1.11 to -0.18) but not late pain (WMD: -0.29, 95% CI: -0.88 to -0.29), and decreased opioid consumption when the 60-mg dose is used, with a difference in mean morphine equivalent dosing of -1.64 mg (95% CI: -2.90 to -0.37 mg). Compared to placebo, there was a greater opioid-sparing effect of ketorolac when intramuscular ketorolac was administered than when intravenous ketorolac was administered, with a difference in mean morphine equivalent dosing of -2.13 mg (95% CI: -4.1 to -0.21 mg). The addition of the 60-mg dose to the analgesic regimen reduced postoperative nausea and vomiting (odds ratio [OR]: 0.49, 95% CI: 0.29-0.81). Unlike the evidence of the effect of a ketorolac 60-mg dose that offers significant benefits in pain relief and opioid-related adverse effects, there is no sufficient evidence to conclude the effect of the 30-mg dose on postoperative pain and opioid outcomes.

Meta-analyses of 5 RCTs ($n = 251$ patients) did not support the lidocaine 5% patch as an adjunct for acute and postoperative pain care in pain intensity (MD: -9.1 mm, 95% CI: -23.31 to 5.20, $Z = 1.24$, $P = 0.21$; $I^2 = 99\%$), opioid consumption (MD: -8.2 mg, 95% CI: -28.68 to 12.24, $Z = 0.79$, $P = 0.43$; $I^2 = 88\%$), and days of hospital stay (MD: -0.2 days, 95% CI: -0.80 to 0.43, $Z = 0.60$, $P = 0.55$; $I^2 = 43\%$), compared to those without the lidocaine patch (Bai, Miller, Tan, Law, & Gan, 2015). Potential biases (e.g., unblinding), heterogeneity (high variability) among studies, and incomplete outcome data on adjunct analgesics remain concerns (Bai et al., 2015).

Zhou, Fan, Zhong, Wen, and Chen (2017) conducted a meta-analysis of 21 RCTs ($n = 1980$ patients) to compare their efficacy and safety of multimodal analgesic approaches to chronic postsurgical pain. The researchers particularly focused on four surgical types, including general, orthopedic, gynecologic, and thoracic. The multimodal anesthesia methods included regional analgesia such as epidural, wound infusion, topical application, plexus blocks, spinal blocks, peritoneal instillation, and paravertebral blocks. Regional analgesia has been shown to be effective in decreasing the frequency of postsurgical pain (relative risk [RR]: 0.69, 95% CI: 0.56-0.85,

$P < 0.001$), with moderate heterogeneity among the included studies ($I^2 = 50.1\%$, $P = 0.007$) and improving overall patient satisfaction (standardized mean difference [SMD]: 1.95, 95% CI: 0.83-3.06, $P = 0.001$), compared to traditional analgesia. No other outcomes were significant, such as opioid consumption, pain rating, functional activity, and mental health inventory. The authors conclude that further research should examine the long-term efficacy and safety of regional analgesic approaches to further verify the current evidence.

In a meta-analysis of 11 RCTs ($n = 899$), use of anticonvulsant (i.e., pregabalin) as an adjunct for perioperative pain management yielded better outcomes, such as a decrease in opioid consumption and vomiting, and mixed results regarding other opioid-related adverse effects including nausea, dizziness and sedation, and headache (Zhang, Ho, & Wang, 2011). No significant difference in pain intensity exists. The use of pregabalin as an adjunct for acute postoperative pain was effective in decreasing cumulative opioid consumption at 24 hours but not pain intensity. A decrease in cumulative opioid consumption depends on pregabalin dosage. At pregabalin doses of less than 300 mg, the opioid-sparing effect was estimated at WMD: 8.8 mg (95% CI: -16.65 to -0.94) and at pregabalin doses 300 mg or more, the opioid-sparing effect was estimated at WMD: 13.40 mg (95% CI: -22.78 to -4.02), with high heterogeneity among the included studies (degrees of freedom $= 2$, $P = 0.007$). Pregabalin had a significant effect on reduction in vomiting (RR: 0.73, 95% CI: 0.56-0.95) but an increased risk of visual disturbance (RR: 3.29, 95% CI: 1.95-5.57). Similarly, meta-analysis of 132 RCTs ($n = 9498$) examined the pooled effects of perioperative gabapentin therapy versus placebo or active placebo on 24-hour opioid use and opioid-related adverse effects (Fabritius et al. 2016). A total of 13 RCTs with low risk of bias found a reduction in 24-hour morphine use of 3.1 mg (95% CI: 0.5-5.6, Trial Sequential Analysis [TSA]-adjusted CI: -0.2 to 6.3). When gabapentin was used as an add-on analgesic to another nonopioid treatment, there was a mean decrease in 24-hour opioid use of 1.2 mg (95% CI: -0.3 to 2.6, TSA-adjusted CI: -0.4 to 2.8) compared to the control group. Nine RCTs with low risk of bias found an RR of serious adverse effects of 1.61 (95% CI: 0.91-2.86, TSA-adjusted CI: 0.57-4.57). However, the interpretation of the results needs caution because of low or very low quality evidence. Strong evidence for the use of gabapentin in perioperative pain care is lacking, and serious adverse effects are forthcoming, particularly when it is added to multimodal regimen.

Murphy et al. (2013) conducted a meta-analysis of 22 RCTs ($n = 1177$) that tested the effect of continuous intravenous magnesium infusions in addition to opioid analgesia on opioid-related outcomes. Patients receiving magnesium demonstrated a significant reduction in morphine use compared to those who only received opioids (WMD: -7.40, 95% CI: -9.40 to -5.41, $P < 0.001$). However, no differences in opioid-related adverse effects exist (RR: 0.76, 95% CI: 0.52-1.09, $P = 0.14$). Patients who received magnesium experienced a significant short-term pain reduction (4-6 hours postsurgery; WMD: -0.67, 95% CI: -1.12 to -0.23, $P = 0.003$) but no longer effect

> ▶ **KEY POINT**
>
> Evidence suggests that multimodal pain management is effective in reducing opioid consumption and opioid-related adverse effects, such as nausea and vomiting, whereas mixed results were noted regarding pain relief in perioperative pain, neck pain, chronic low back pain, fibromyalgia, and cancer pain.

(20-24 hours postsurgery; WMD: -0.25, 95% CI: -0.62 to 0.71, $P = 0.17$) compared to those without magnesium infusions. The authors concluded that perioperative intravenous magnesium infusions can be a useful addition to opioids for postoperative pain management but were not associated with a reduction in opioid-related adverse effects.

Meta-analysis of 14 RCTs ($n = 713$ patients) did not support the combination of tramadol and morphine among adult surgical patients regarding pain intensity and opioid-related adverse effects, whereas it supported a limited but significant opioid-sparing effect with an WMD of 6.9 mg (95% CI: -11.3 to -2.5; Martinez, Guichard, & Fletcher, 2015).

Neck Pain

A meta-analysis of 33 RCTs by Leaver, Refshauge, Maher, and McAuley (2010) was conducted to test the effects of conservative interventions on pain intensity and disability among individuals with nonspecific neck pain. Among 33 RCTs, 2 unique studies compared multimodal physical therapies such as exercise, massage, and various electrotherapies, with minimal intervention including advice on simple, regular exercises (Hoving et al., 2002, 2006; Palmgren, Sandstrom, Lundqvist, & Heikkila, 2006). Multimodal physical therapy including spinal manual therapy had a significant improvement in pain posttreatment (MD: -21, 95% CI: -34 to -7) but no long-term pain and disability outcomes (Palmgren et al., 2006). Multimodal physical therapy without manual therapy yielded no difference in pain and disability outcomes compared to a control group upon completion of treatment at both the medium and long term (Hoving et al., 2002, 2006).

Low Back Pain

A Cochrane review of 9 RCTs ($n = 981$ participants) was conducted on multidisciplinary biopsychosocial rehabilitation programs targeting the multifaceted nature of pain, administered by professionals from diverse disciplines (Marin et al., 2017). Compared to individuals with subacute low back pain receiving usual care, those who receive multidisciplinary biopsychosocial rehabilitation had less pain (SMD: -0.46, 95% CI: -0.70 to -0.21) in 4 studies ($n = 336$), less disability (SMD: -0.44, 95% CI: -0.87 to -0.01) in 3 studies ($n = 240$), fewer sick days (SMD: -0.38, 95% CI: -0.66 to -0.10) in 2 studies ($n = 210$), and were more likely to return to work at 1 year follow-up (OR: 3.19, 95% CI: 1.46-6.98) in 3 studies ($n = 170$). In terms of clinical significance, the authors noted that work-related outcomes tend to have moderate effect sizes, whereas pain and disability had low effect sizes. However, there was no between-group difference in pain in 2 studies ($n = 336$; SMD: -0.14, 95% CI: -0.36 to 0.07), functional disability in 2 studies ($n = 345$; SMD: -0.03, 95% CI: -0.24 to 0.18), and time away from work in 2 studies ($n = 158$) when compared to other types of intervention, such as brief interventions including education and advice on physical activity. None of these studies reported return to work as an outcome variable. It should be noted that available studies provide very low quality to low-quality evidence.

A meta-analysis of 24 RCTs that followed up with participants at 12 weeks postintervention was conducted to determine the pooled effect of conservative interventions including physical, behavioral, and combined interventions on chronic low back pain management (O'Keeffe et al., 2016). The results generally presented low effect sizes for pain intensity at short-term (5 studies, $n = 529$; MD: 0.52, 95% CI: 0.16-0.88, $I^2 = 4\%$) and long-term (15 studies, $n = 1453$; MD: 0.47, 95% CI: 0.13-0.81, $I^2 = 35\%$) follow-ups and disability at short-term (5 studies, $n = 529$; SMD: 0.27, 95% CI: 0.01-0.54, $I^2 = 56\%$) and long-term (13 studies, $n = 1189$; SMD: 0.25, 95% CI: 0.07-0.43, $I^2 = 54\%$) follow-ups when the combined interventions were compared to physical intervention. However, the results have not reached clinical significance. The authors also noted that the simple categorization of each intervention into three groups might have affected the pooled results because of the difficulty differentiating the original purpose of these interventions.

Chronic Pain Conditions

Dragioti, Evangelou, Larsson, and Gerdle (2018) conducted an umbrella review of 12 meta-analyses and 24 qualitative systematic reviews to determine if multidisciplinary rehabilitation programs were effective in promoting pain-related outcomes compared to other active or inactive conditions. Multidisciplinary rehabilitation programs were defined as an intervention that includes at least two distinct components, such as 1+ physical and 1+ psychological therapy or educational component. The authors conclude that there was no strong or highly suggestive evidence that multidisciplinary rehabilitation programs are effective in managing common pain conditions such as lower back pain, neck pain, and fibromyalgia. The nonsignificant findings were likely associated with the included associations between interventions and outcomes solely for low back pain, predominantly regarding short-term effects.

Cancer Pain

A subgroup analysis (7 RCTs; $n = 437$) of the meta-analysis of 15 RCTs ($n = 1157$) supported acupuncture as an adjunct to conventional drug therapy for cancer pain (Choi, Lee, Kim, Zaslawski, & Ernst, 2012). Acupuncture with conventional drug treatment on cancer pain versus drug therapy alone showed favorable effects of acupuncture on pain relief (RR: 1.36, 95% CI: 1.13-1.64, $P = 0.003$) with high heterogeneity ($\chi^2 = 19.92$, $P = 0.003$, $I^2 = 70\%$). However, in a subgroup analysis of this meta-analysis (8 studies; $n = 886$), acupuncture did not show a superior effect on cancer pain over drug therapy (RR: 1.12, 95% CI: 0.98-1.28, $P = 0.09$).

Chen, Li, Cho, and Zhang (2013) examined the impact of acupoint stimulation as an adjunct treatment for lung cancer on cancer pain control, functional status, immediate tumor response, and quality of life. Those who received acupoint simulation plus other active treatment had a significant improvement in $CD3^+$ T-cell level in 9 studies ($n = 370$; SMD: 0.41, 95% CI: 0.20-0.62, $P = 0.0001$) and $CD4^+$ T-cell level in 10 studies ($n = 459$; SMD: 0.61, 95% CI: 0.42-0.80, $P < 0.00001$) compared to those who received other active treatments. The acupoint stimulation group demonstrated a significant reduction in the frequency of chemotherapy-induced nausea and vomiting at Grade II toIV compared to the control group in 8 studies ($n = 501$; RR: 0.46, 95% CI: 0.37-0.51, $P < 0.001$). A subgroup analysis showed that needle insertion, injection with herbs, and moxibustion significantly diminished the magnitude of nausea and vomiting ($P = 0.02$, 0.005, and 0.01, respectively). In 2 studies ($n = 85$), the acupoint stimulation group plus other therapy showed a favorable effect on quality of life compared to other therapies alone (SMD: 0.47, 95% CI: 0.04-0.90, $P = 0.03$). In addition, a significant reduction in pain score was witnessed in the acupoint stimulation group compared to the control group in 2 studies ($n = 92$; SMD: -1.13, 95% CI: -1.58 to -0.69, $P < 0.001$).

▌ Fibromyalgia

Papadopoulou, Fassoulaki, Tsoulas, Siafaka, and Vadalouca (2016) conducted a meta-analysis of 46 RCTs with pharmacologic and 77 RCTs with nonpharmacologic agents, and 2 each of pharmacologic and nonpharmacologic arms. The control group included drug, placebo or sham intervention, waiting list, treatment as usual, or standard of care. The authors found that nonpharmacologic multidisciplinary care was more effective in reducing pain in 7 studies ($n = 703$; effect size [ES]: -0.42, 95% CI: -0.59 to -0.24), improving sleep in 5 studies ($n = 478$; ES: -0.44, 95% CI: -0.63 to -0.26), increasing function in 5 studies ($n = 469$; ES: -0.37, 95% CI: -0.61 to -0.13), decreasing fatigue in 5 studies ($n = 469$; ES: -0.35, 95% CI: -0.58 to -0.12), lowering anxiety in 5 studies ($n = 470$; ES: -0.33, 95% CI: -0.59 to -0.06), and decreasing depression in 5 studies ($n = 632$; ES: -0.33, 95% CI: -0.64 to -0.02). However, the magnitude of the effect size tended to be small. These findings are consistent with a subgroup analysis of another meta-analysis of 102 RCTs that originally compared the efficacy of pharmacologic and nonpharmacologic intervention in fibromyalgia (Nuesch, Hauser, Bernardy, Barth, & Juni, 2013). Of the 102 RCTs included in this meta-analysis, 15 RCTs ($n = 1751$) focused on multicomponent therapy. The pooled results were calculated for studies that are of medium size (>50 patients per group) and showed a small to moderate effect size over the placebo regarding pain (SMD: -0.47, 95% CI: -0.69 to -0.24) and quality of life (SMD: -0.56, 95% CI: -0.76 to -0.36; Nuesch et al., 2013).

▌ Other Musculoskeletal Pain

Meta-analysis of 27 RCTs supported the multimodal physiotherapy in the short term but not at 6, 12, or 52 weeks regarding pain reduction in cases of anterior knee care (Collins, Bisset, Crossley, & Vicenzino, 2012). From 27 studies, the result from a meta-analysis of 2 RCTs showed a moderate effect of multimodal physiotherapy over a placebo treatment at 6 weeks in cases of anterior knee pain (SMD: 1.08, 95% CI: 0.73-1.143; Collins et al., 2008; Crossley, Bennell, Green, Cowan, & McConnell, 2002). In one study measuring the mid- and long-term effects of pain reduction methods (Collins et al., 2008), the effect was attenuated at 12 weeks (SMD: 0.69, 95% CI: 0.23-1.14), and a small effect was witnessed at 1 year (SMD: 0.44, 95% CI: 0.01-0.88). When compared to other nonsurgical treatments, multimodal physiotherapy produced small to moderate effect sizes. However, the magnitude of the effect size was attenuated at long-term follow-up (e.g., 1 year). Collins et al. (2008) also observed a small effect size of multimodal physiotherapy versus foot orthoses on anterior knee pain at 6 weeks (SMD: 0.51, 95% CI: 0.07, 0.95) and 12 weeks (SMD: 0.45, 95% CI: 0.01-0.88), but not at 1 year. Furthermore, in the study (Collins et al., 2008), when multimodal physiotherapy was used as an adjunct to foot orthoses compared to foot orthoses alone, the study produced a moderate effect at all time points over 1 year (6 weeks: SMD 0.87, 95% CI: 0.42-1.32; 12 weeks: SMD: 0.63, 95% CI: 0.16-1.07; 52 weeks: SMD: 0.70, 95% CI: 0.27-1.14).

Shoulder Hand Syndrome

Meta-analysis of 20 RCTs ($n = 1918$) supported traditional manual acupuncture plus rehabilitation therapy for shoulder hand syndrome care after stroke compared to rehabilitation therapy alone (Peng et al., 2018). The combined therapy yielded reduction in pain (MD: 1.49, 95% CI: 1.15-1.82, $P < 0.001$) with severe heterogeneity ($I^2 = 71\%$, $P = 0.0005$), improvement in lower extremity movement (MD: 8.42, 95% CI: 6.74-10.10, $P < 0.00001$) with severe heterogeneity ($I^2 = 94\%$, $P < 0.00001$), and activities of daily living (SMD: 1.31, 95% CI: 0.57-2.05, $P = 0.0005$) with high heterogeneity ($I^2 = 95\%$, $P < 0.00001$) compared to rehabilitation therapy alone. However, the results should be interpreted with caution because of their high variability.

Conclusion

Multimodal pain management is considered a logical management approach to targeting the biologic, psychological, and social components affecting pain. A growing number of studies have supported the claim that multimodal pain management is generally effective in promoting functional activity and reducing opioid consumption and opioid-related adverse effects, including vomiting and nausea, in individuals with certain pain conditions (perioperative pain, low back pain, and fibromyalgia). However, the pooled results should be interpreted with caution because of the high variability of the included studies and the difficulty differentiating the classification of intervention components such as physical, psychological, and social components. Current evidence predominantly focuses on perioperative multimodal analgesia, including the limited literature on lower back pain. In addition, this chapter includes the results from meta-analyses that were written in English and were found in one electronic database (i.e., PubMed), published before January 2019. With pain research evolving with an emphasis on a personalized approach to pain management, multimodal pain management is one of the promising avenues for improving quality of life among individuals with pain conditions. However, more research with high methodological rigor that targets different aspects of multidimensional of pain should be conducted to produce high-quality evidence.

REFERENCES

Bai, Y., Miller, T., Tan, M., Law, L. S., & Gan, T. J. (2015). Lidocaine patch for acute pain management: A meta-analysis of prospective controlled trials. *Current Medical Research and Opinion, 31*(3), 575–581. doi:10.1185/03007995.2014.973484

Chen, H. Y., Li, S. G., Cho, W. C., & Zhang, Z. J. (2013). The role of acupoint stimulation as an adjunct therapy for lung cancer: A systematic review and meta-analysis. *BMC Complementary and Alternative Medicine, 13*, 362. doi:10.1186/1472-6882-13-362

Choi, T. Y., Lee, M. S., Kim, T. H., Zaslawski, C., & Ernst, E. (2012). Acupuncture for the treatment of cancer pain: A systematic review of randomised clinical trials. *Supportive Care in Cancer, 20*(6), 1147–1158. doi:10.1007/s00520-012-1432-9

Chou, R., Gordon, D. B., de Leon-Casasola, O. A., Rosenberg, J. M., Bickler, S., Brennan, T., . . . Wu, C. L. (2016). Management of postoperative pain: A Clinical Practice Guideline From the American Pain Society, the American Society of Regional Anesthesia and Pain Medicine, and the American Society of Anesthesiologists' Committee on Regional Anesthesia, Executive Committee, and Administrative Council. *Journal of Pain, 17*(2), 131–157. doi:10.1016/j.jpain.2015.12.008

Collins, N. J., Bisset, L. M., Crossley, K. M., & Vicenzino, B. (2012). Efficacy of nonsurgical interventions for anterior knee pain: Systematic review and meta-analysis of randomized trials. *Sports Medicine, 42*(1), 31–49. doi:10.2165/11594460-000000000-00000

Collins, N., Crossley, K., Beller, E., Darnell, R., McPoil, T., & Vicenzino, B. (2008). Foot orthoses and physiotherapy in the treatment of patellofemoral pain syndrome: Randomised clinical trial. *BMJ, 337*, a1735. doi:10.1136/bmj.a1735

Crossley, K., Bennell, K., Green, S., Cowan, S., & McConnell, J. (2002). Physical therapy for patellofemoral pain: A randomized, double-blinded, placebo-controlled trial. *American Journal of Sports Medicine, 30*(6), 857–865. doi:10.1177/03635465020300061701

De Oliveira, G. S., Jr., Agarwal, D., & Benzon, H. T. (2012). Perioperative single dose ketorolac to prevent postoperative pain: A meta-analysis of randomized trials. *Anesthesia & Analgesia, 114*(2), 424–433. doi:10.1213/ANE.0b013e3182334d68

Department of Health and Human Services. (2016). *National pain strategy: A comprehensive population health strategy for pain*. Retrieved from https://iprcc.nih.gov/sites/default/files/HHSNational_Pain_Strategy_508C.pdf

Dragioti, E., Evangelou, E., Larsson, B., & Gerdle, B. (2018). Effectiveness of multidisciplinary programmes for clinical pain conditions: An umbrella review. *Journal of Rehabilitation Medicine, 50*(9), 779–791. doi:10.2340/16501977-2377

Fabritius, M. L., Geisler, A., Petersen, P. L., Nikolajsen, L., Hansen, M. S., Kontinen, V., . . . Mathiesen, O. (2016). Gabapentin for post-operative pain management—A systematic review with meta-analyses and trial sequential analyses. *Acta Anaesthesiologica Scandinavica, 60*(9), 1188–1208. doi:10.1111/aas.12766

Gatchel, R. J. (2005). *Clinical essentials of pain management*. Washington DC: American Psychological Association.

Gatchel, R. J., Peng, Y. B., Peters, M. L., Fuchs, P. N., & Turk, D. C. (2007). The biopsychosocial approach to chronic pain: Scientific advances and future directions. *Psychological Bulletin, 133*(4), 581–624. doi:10.1037/0033-2909.133.4.581

Hoving, J. L., de Vet, H. C., Koes, B. W., Mameren, H., Deville, W. L., van der Windt, D. A., . . . Bouter, L. M. (2006). Manual therapy, physical therapy, or continued care by the general practitioner for patients with neck pain: Long-term results from a pragmatic randomized clinical trial. *Clinical Journal of Pain, 22*(4), 370–377. doi:10.1097/01.ajp.0000180185.79382.3f

Hoving, J. L., Koes, B. W., de Vet, H. C., van der Windt, D. A., Assendelft, W. J., van Mameren, H., . . . Bouter, L. M. (2002). Manual therapy, physical therapy, or continued care by a general practitioner for patients with neck pain. A randomized, controlled trial. *Annals of Internal Medicine, 136*(10), 713–722.

Institute of Medicine. (2011). *Relieving pain in America: A blueprint for transforming prevention, care, education, and research*. Washington, DC: The National Academices Press.

International Association for the Study of Pain. (1994). Part III: Pain terms, a current list with definitions and notes on usage. In H. Merskey & N. Bogduk (Eds.), *Classification of chronic pain* (IASP task force on taxonomy, IASP terminology, 2nd ed., pp. 209–214). Seattle, WA: Author.

Leaver, A. M., Refshauge, K. M., Maher, C. G., & McAuley, J. H. (2010). Conservative interventions provide short-term relief for non-specific neck pain: A systematic review. *Journal of Physiotherapy, 56*(2), 73–85.

Manworren, R. C. (2015). Multimodal pain management and the future of a personalized medicine approach to pain. *Association of Operating Room Nurses Journal, 101*(3), 308–314; quiz 315–318. doi:10.1016/j.aorn.2014.12.009

Marin, T. J., Van Eerd, D., Irvin, E., Couban, R., Koes, B. W., Malmivaara, A., . . . Kamper, S. J. (2017). Multidisciplinary biopsychosocial rehabilitation for subacute low back pain. *Cochrane Database of Systematic Reviews, 6*, CD002193. doi:10.1002/14651858.CD002193.pub2

Martinez, V., Guichard, L., & Fletcher, D. (2015). Effect of combining tramadol and morphine in adult surgical patients: A systematic review and meta-analysis of randomized trials. *British Journal of Anaesthesia, 114*(3), 384–395. doi:10.1093/bja/aeu414

Muller-Schwefe, G., Morlion, B., Ahlbeck, K., Alon, E., Coaccioli, S., Coluzzi, F., . . . Sichere, P. (2017). Treatment for chronic low back pain: The focus should change to multimodal management that reflects the underlying pain mechanisms. *Current Medical Research and Opinion, 33*(7), 1199–1210. doi:10.1080/03007995.2017.1298521

Murphy, J. D., Paskaradevan, J., Eisler, L. L., Ouanes, J. P., Tomas, V. A., Freck, E. A., & Wu, C. L. (2013). Analgesic efficacy of continuous intravenous magnesium infusion as an adjuvant to morphine for postoperative analgesia: A systematic review and meta-analysis. *Middle East Journal of Anaesthesiology, 22*(1), 11–20.

Nuesch, E., Hauser, W., Bernardy, K., Barth, J., & Juni, P. (2013). Comparative efficacy of pharmacological and non-pharmacological interventions in fibromyalgia syndrome: Network meta-analysis. *Annals of the Rheumatic Diseases, 72*(6), 955–962. doi:10.1136/annrheumdis-2011-201249

O'Keeffe, M., Purtill, H., Kennedy, N., Conneely, M., Hurley, J., O'Sullivan, P., . . . O'Sullivan, K. (2016). Comparative effectiveness of conservative interventions for nonspecific chronic spinal pain: Physical, behavioral/psychological informed, or combined? A systematic review and meta-analysis. *Journal of Pain, 17*(7), 755–774. doi:10.1016/j.jpain.2016.01.473

Palmgren, P. J., Sandstrom, P. J., Lundqvist, F. J., & Heikkila, H. (2006). Improvement after chiropractic care in cervicocephalic kinesthetic sensibility and subjective pain intensity in patients with nontraumatic chronic neck pain. *Journal of Manipulative and Physiological Therapeutics, 29*(2), 100–106. doi:10.1016/j.jmpt.2005.12.002

Papadopoulou, D., Fassoulaki, A., Tsoulas, C., Siafaka, I., & Vadalouca, A. (2016). A meta-analysis to determine the effect of pharmacological and non-pharmacological treatments on fibromyalgia symptoms comprising OMERACT-10 response criteria. *Clinical Rheumatology, 35*(3), 573–586. doi:10.1007/s10067-015-3144-2

Peng, L., Zhang, C., Zhou, L., Zuo, H. X., He, X. K., & Niu, Y. M. (2018). Traditional manual acupuncture combined with rehabilitation therapy for shoulder hand syndrome after stroke within the Chinese healthcare system: A systematic review and meta-analysis. *Clinical Rehabilitation, 32*(4), 429–439. doi:10.1177/0269215517729528

Zhang, J., Ho, K. Y., & Wang, Y. (2011). Efficacy of pregabalin in acute postoperative pain: A meta-analysis. *British Journal of Anaesthesia, 106*(4), 454–462. doi:10.1093/bja/aer027

Zhou, J., Fan, Y., Zhong, J., Wen, X., & Chen, H. (2017). Efficacy and safety of multimodal analgesic techniques for preventing chronic postsurgery pain under different surgical categories: A meta-analysis. *Scientific Reports, 7*(1), 678. doi:10.1038/s41598-017-00813-5

CHAPTER 6

PSYCHOTHERAPY AND COGNITIVE-BEHAVIORAL THERAPY

Jessica W. Guite and Michael Reiss

▌Introduction

With the advent of the biopsychosocial model of pain (Engel, 1977), there is a greater appreciation of the role that factors such as emotion, cognition, and social interaction can play in the experience of pain. Because pain is defined as a "mutually recognizable somatic experience that reflects a person's apprehension of threat to their bodily or existential integrity" (Cohen, Quintner, & van Rysewyk, 2018), it is also amenable to interventions that impact these factors. The majority of psychotherapy research focusing on chronic pain has examined cognitive-behavioral therapy (CBT). CBT was originally developed by Aaron Beck, MD in the 1960s (Beck, 1963) to treat depression, and it differed from other psychotherapies (e.g., psychodynamic and behavioral) of the time (Strupp & Binder, 1984; Wolpe, 1973). CBT emphasizes the modification of dysfunctional thinking in order to bring about lasting emotional and behavioral change (Beck, 2011; Beck, Rush, Shaw, & Emery, 1979). It is a model-driven approach that is structured, can be readily taught, can be empirically assessed, and has an emphasis on solving present problems within a relatively short period of time and therapeutic contacts.

More recent developments, referred to as the "third wave" of CBT, include interventions such as acceptance and commitment therapy (ACT), dialectic behavior therapy, functional analytic psychotherapy, mindfulness-based cognitive therapy, and other acceptance- and mindfulness-based approaches. Of these, ACT has been among the most frequently used for patients with chronic pain. ACT was developed by Steven Hayes, PhD and incorporates acceptance and mindfulness strategies to change a person's relationship with and perspective on psychological events in order to gain psychological flexibility and engage in committed action (Hayes, Pistorello, & Levin, 2012; Hayes, Strosahl, & Wilson, 1999). Both CBT and ACT have been adapted for use with patients with chronic pain, with research to support the efficacy of psychotherapeutic interventions for patients coping with chronic pain conditions throughout development.

Evidence for Psychotherapy Interventions for Chronic Pain

The critically important role of psychosocial factors within biopsychosocial approaches to treatment is well supported by evidence for the benefits of psychotherapy to treat children, adolescents, and adults with chronic pain. We provide a brief review of the evidence base for psychotherapy to treat children and adolescents with chronic pain followed by research with adults with chronic pain.

Children and Adolescents

There has been recent evidence supporting the use of psychotherapy to treat chronic pain in children and adolescents. Eccleston et al.'s (2014) systematic review of 37 randomized controlled trials for the management of chronic and recurrent pain in children and adolescents found that psychological treatments tended to be behavioral or cognitive behavioral. The majority of research in Eccleston et al.'s review has been done on youth with headaches ($n = 20/37$). This review found that psychological treatment was effective in reducing pain intensity and disability in children with chronic headache with lasting effects, although the sample size was small. For children and adolescents with other chronic pain conditions besides headache ($n = 17/37$ studies), there is evidence to support reduced pain outcomes immediately posttreatment (but not evidence to support maintenance of gains at follow-up for those with mixed pain [i.e., both headache and nonheadache pain]). Results of this systematic review of available research also provide evidence for the effectiveness of relaxation and CBT for reducing pain intensity in children with headache, abdominal pain, fibromyalgia, and sickle cell disease when assessed immediately posttreatment. It was concluded that 56% of children treated with psychological therapies reported less pain, compared to 22% of children not receiving therapy. A related meta-analysis closely examined the benefits of psychotherapy and explored optimal dose of treatment for pediatric chronic pain conditions including headache, abdominal, musculoskeletal, and neuropathic pain (Fisher et al., 2014). Results examined outcomes for pain, disability, depression, anxiety, and sleep. Psychotherapy for headache pain improved symptoms significantly at posttreatment and at follow-up, with higher treatment dose leading to greater reductions in pain. For abdominal pain, significant improvements in pain and disability were found, whereas children experiencing musculoskeletal pain had significantly reduced pain, disability, and depression posttreatment, which was sustained for disability at follow-up.

Adults

There is similar evidence to support the efficacy of psychotherapy treatment for adults with chronic pain. Williams, Eccleston, and Morley (2012) examined 35 randomized controlled trials comparing psychological therapy (CBT and behavior therapy) with control conditions (either waitlist or treatment as usual). They found that CBT had small positive effects on disability and catastrophizing, but not on pain or mood, in comparison to control conditions. Pain, disability, mood, and catastrophizing improved immediately posttreatment compared to controls, with a small effect for improvement in mood maintained at follow-up. The authors noted that there is an absence of evidence for behavioral therapy, which tends to be focused solely on increasing desirable behaviors, with less focus on thoughts and feelings (Wolpe, 1973). Bernardy, Klose, Busch, Choy, and Häuser's (2013) systematic review found similar benefits of treating fibromyalgia with CBT. Specifically, they found that CBT slightly reduces pain, negative mood, and disability in children, adolescents, and adults immediately after treatment and at 6-month follow-up. Although there is widespread support for the benefits of CBT for many chronic pain conditions, Eccleston, Hearn, and Williams' (2015) review of psychological treatment for chronic neuropathic pain in adults did not find clear benefit of psychological treatment for all neuropathic conditions (e.g., spinal cord injury and burning mouth syndrome).

The literature also shows evidence for beneficial effects of treating adult chronic pain with ACT. Hughes, Clark, Colclough, Dale, and McMillan (2017) examined 11 randomized controlled trials comparing ACT to a control condition, active treatment, or waitlist/active treatment. They found significant, medium to large effect sizes for outcomes including pain acceptance and psychological flexibility. Small to medium effect sizes were found for outcomes including improved physical functioning, anxiety, and depression; however, no significant effects were found for quality of life and pain intensity. Stability of these findings at follow-up tended to show smaller effect sizes. It is important to interpret these findings in the context of the current limited number of trials examining ACT or that compare ACT to other active treatments. Although ACT treatments presently show promising short-term initial improvement for outcomes, the stability of these findings over time is diminished.

Conclusion

There is evidence to support that using CBT to treat chronic pain is beneficial both in children and in adults. The most compelling evidence in support of CBT focuses primarily on reduction of pain intensity and disability for both children and adults experiencing chronic pain immediately postintervention. Additional research to support CBT's beneficial effect on pain and disability (and related outcomes) at long-term follow-up is needed. Although benefits of CBT are generally appreciated by interdisciplinary clinicians working in busy medical settings, questions remain as to when and how best to refer patients to participate in this treatment. Consideration of these questions will be a focus of the following sections.

Chronic Pain and Associated Mental Health Concerns

Many patients with chronic pain experience pain-related anxiety, also termed pain "catastrophizing," which has been described as "an exaggerated negative orientation toward noxious stimuli" (Sullivan, Bishop, & Pivik, 1995, p. 524). Tunks, Crook, and Weir's (2008) overview of the epidemiology of chronic pain illustrates how chronic pain significantly predicts new onset of depression and that

> ▶ **KEY POINT**
>
> When an individual has been in pain for longer than 3 months, the persistence of this problem and the need for sustained coping become a source of stress unto itself. There are psychological symptoms and behaviors that are frequently, but not always, associated with chronic pain including anxiety, depression, sleep problems, substance use, and eating disorders.

depression significantly predicts the onset of chronic pain among adult samples. Similarly, among a nationally representative cohort of adolescents, Tegethoff, Belardi, Stalujanis, and Meinlschmidt (2015) found approximately 25% of the sample experienced chronic pain and mental disorder in their lifetime on the World Health Organization Composite International Diagnostic Interview Version 3.0 (World Health Organization, 2018). The co-occurrence of chronic pain and mental disorders for teenagers ranged from 1.91% for presence of any eating disorder to 17.40% for presence of any anxiety disorder. The authors found that anxiety, affective, and behavior disorders may be risk factors for chronic pain.

In addition to these mental disorders associated with chronic pain, there is growing consensus of a relationship with adverse childhood experiences (ACEs) (e.g., physical abuse, sexual abuse, early parental loss). ACEs may alter the hypothalamus-pituitary-adrenal axis, in turn putting an exposed individual at risk for mental disorder and pain-related issues (Felitti et al., 1998). Sachs-Ericsson, Sheffler, Stanley, Piazza, and Preacher's (2017) longitudinal study found that verbal and sexual abuse, early parental loss, and parent psychopathology were associated with painful medical issues. Nelson, Simons, and Logan (2018) found that 82% of youth with chronic pain report at least one ACE in their lifetime, with almost one-fourth having three or more ACEs, and that ACE exposure was significantly associated with psychological distress (e.g., anxiety, depression). Salazar et al.'s (2013) retrospective cohort study of over 1000 adults in primary care with musculoskeletal pain found a high level of undiagnosed mood disorders, with female gender, high pain intensity, and sleep disruption because of pain contributing to this diagnosis. Apart from distinct mental illness, chronic pain inevitably raises levels of stress, which tends to exacerbate pain levels. One cannot underestimate the contribution of psychological factors to a patient's experience with chronic pain.

When to Refer a Patient with Chronic Pain to Therapy

When a patient experiences pain for 3 months or longer, functional limitations that were not present before the onset of pain are more likely to occur (Bursch, Walco, & Zeltzer, 1998). This section reviews functional limitations that are common to people experiencing chronic pain. In addition, we will consider the value of referring a patient with chronic pain and disability for psychological intervention to facilitate increasing engagement in treatment recommendations (e.g., physical therapy adherence) or address psychosocial factors that serve to impede engagement in functional activities.

Children and Adolescents

When a child or adolescent experiences chronic pain, school performance, peer relationships, sleep, family functioning, and physical activity are often disrupted (Palermo, 2012). As noted earlier, trauma (i.e., ACEs) and pain can be highly comorbid, which can further contribute to disability and ripple effects that radiate across systems of support (Guite, Logan, Ely, & Weisman, 2012). For example, children and adolescents may experience declining school attendance and associated declining grades. Chronic pain may also interfere with peer relationships, especially if the child is not attending school and is isolated from others. Sleep may also be disrupted because of chronic pain. It is important to note that sleep and chronic pain have been shown to have a bidirectional relationship (McCracken & Iverson, 2002) and that complex patterns of parent-child interactions have also been implicated in the associations among sleep, pain, and disability (Puzino, Guite, Moore, Lewen, & Williamson, 2017). Chronic pain affects not just the individual, but the family as well (Jordan, Eccleston, & Osborn, 2007; Palermo & Chambers, 2005).

Relationships are prone to change as caregivers can check in more with a child or adolescent giving way to an enmeshed relational style, which may further set the child back. Parent caregivers may respond differently to a child or adolescent's pain, which may create further familial conflict. Finally, physical activity limited by chronic pain can disengage children and adolescents from participating in previously pleasurable activities, which may also impact the social domain.

> **▶ KEY POINT**
>
> It is advisable for clinicians to routinely assess chronic pain and its associated disability in a standardized and validated manner over time.

The Functional Disability Inventory (Walker & Greene, 1991) is a valid and reliable instrument for children 8 to 18 years of age with chronic or recurrent pain that can be of help to understand a child's current functioning and limitations across several domains as well as provide a window into the response to treatment over time. Measures such as the National Institutes of Health (NIH) Patient-Reported Outcomes Measurement Information System (PROMIS) (Cella et al., 2007; Kashikar-Zuck, Carle, et al., 2016), as well as multiple other brief, validated measures are freely available to facilitate assessment for both children and adults seen in clinical settings (Beidas et al., 2015). Consensus recommendations for selection of outcome measures for clinical trials focusing on pediatric chronic pain have also been provided (McGrath et al., 2008).

▌ Adults

Functional disability for adults with chronic pain has many similarities to children with respect to physical and social domains. Whereas youth with chronic pain often experience disruption in school attendance (i.e., their primary vocation/responsibility), chronic pain for adults can significantly impact an adult's occupational functioning (Gatchel, 2004), such as the ability to work inside or outside the home. This may impact earning potential (Anagnostis, Gatchel, & Mayer, 2004) and can place added strain on relationships with significant others, especially if they are interdependent on others (e.g., spouses) for financial and emotional support. Deficits in activities of daily living (e.g., grasping for objects and personal care) may be pronounced for adults with chronic pain. The NIH PROMIS (Cella et al., 2007) provides brief, validated measures for the assessment of pain, disability, and various emotional factors frequently co-occurring with chronic pain. Various other specialized legacy measures have been developed and validated within specific chronic pain populations, with consensus recommendations for selection of outcome measures for clinical trials also provided (Dworkin et al., 2005; Turk et al., 2006).

Prerequisite Skills Needed to Refer and Apply CBT

Providers are encouraged to discuss the potential for referral for behavioral health support for patients with chronic pain at the first care contact. The importance of setting the stage for clear and open communication about the benefits of behavioral health support and evidence for CBT efficacy in the treatment of chronic pain cannot be understated (Guite et al., 2012, 2014). Commitment to a biopsychosocial approach to pain management that dispels mind-body dualistic thinking aids providers in taking an educational stance with their patients about the important role that CBT can play in a pain coping toolkit. Providers need to appreciate that patients and families often may be reluctant to initially raise questions about this treatment modality because of concerns about stigma or worry that providers do not believe the pain is "real" and won't help them unless there is a "biologic" underpinning for the pain symptoms. Having established open communication about the important role that behavioral health plays in pain coping early on, making a referral for these services when indicated becomes quite smooth and straightforward. The emphasis of this section is twofold: suggestions for how to initiate and complete a successful psychological referral and how to set the stage for a patient/family to successfully engage in treatment.

> ▶ **KEY POINT**
>
> A discussion of the biopsychosocial approach will be imperative to ensure that the patient understanding of their pain is accurate and they can see the utility of psychological intervention. It will also be important to elicit their beliefs about psychotherapy and what they understand about this intervention.

Understanding the Patient Perception of Pain and Psychotherapy

A patient who has exhibited pain for 3 months or longer has likely been to several different medical providers and may have come away (or been told) in the process that there is little direct medical explanation for their pain and that the pain is all "in their head." Patients tend to internalize such experiences from prior visits, which can directly impact present care. Patients may have a negative view of the medical care and associated psychological recommendations they have received prior to the visit. Before referring a patient with chronic pain for therapy, one must be careful to listen to and validate patient experiences. What have other providers told them about their pain and how can therapy be beneficial? It is not uncommon for individuals with chronic pain to exhibit stigma in the medical setting, especially because chronic pain is often invisible to others and complex in nature (Collier, 2018).

The Therapeutic Alliance

The therapeutic alliance is the bedrock in the relationship between the patient and the provider and has been described as representing mutual collaboration and partnership between the patient and the therapist (Horvath, Del Re, Flückiger, & Symonds, 2011). Rogers' (1957) seminal paper describes that the necessary and sufficient conditions of therapeutic personality change that transcends strictly "psychotherapeutic" relationships include empathy (sensing the client's world as one's own), congruence (genuineness), and unconditional positive regard (warmly accepting the patient). Horvath et al.'s (2011) meta-analysis found a moderate and highly reliable association between alliance and psychotherapeutic outcome. More recently, Welmers-van de Poll et al.'s (2018) meta-analysis of alliance in treatment outcome of youth participating in family involved treatment found that quality of alliance was significantly associated with treatment outcome.

Active Listening

Active listening is one way to engage the patient in order to foster and build the therapeutic alliance. It requires the provider to listen for total meaning both in content and feeling through acknowledgment of the patient's experience (Rogers & Farson, 1987). Just by listening, a provider can ensure that the patient feels heard and conveys that one cares about the patient and demonstrates respect for them. This is especially important for patients with chronic pain who may have been followed by multiple providers with varying levels of alliance with each provider. How does a patient know that you are listening? Exhibiting nonverbal signals such as nodding and making eye contact can be helpful in this regard. Verbally, the clinician can reflect or rephrase what they hear from the patient to ensure they are understanding what the patient is saying. Active listening and reflection can lead to an enhanced therapeutic alliance and a greater shared understanding between the patient and clinician and provide critically important opportunities for providers to dispel misunderstandings or misconceptions that may otherwise sabotage desired treatment goals. With the advent of the electronic health record, the clinician needs to balance not only attention to documentation but also attention to the patient to ensure optimal engagement (Sulmasy, López, Horwitch, American College of Physicians Ethics, & Professionalism Human Rights Committee, 2017).

> ▶ **KEY POINT**
>
> When treating an individual with chronic pain, the therapeutic alliance is of utmost importance and may have been lacking for patients in prior relationships with providers. Thus, providers may need to invest time in providing patients/families with education around the biopsychosocial model of pain to build a foundation for engagement in following up on any recommendation made.

Motivational Interviewing and Establishing a Patient's Readiness to Change

Miller and Rollnick (2012) developed and created motivational interviewing (MI) in order to decrease ambivalence related to behavior change via strengthening a patient's motivation to change. Alperstein and Sharpe's (2016) meta-analysis to better understand the efficacy of MI in adults experiencing chronic pain found that MI can increase short-term adherence to treatment for chronic pain but did not show gains in physical function compared to controls. Patients with chronic pain may have some ambivalence about modifying their lifestyle in order to manage their pain. Eliciting the pros and cons of making versus not making changes can help the clinician understand the patient's ambivalence and increase motivation to change. Most of the literature for MI and chronic pain focuses on adults. Chilton, Pires-Yfantouda, and Wylie's (2012) systematic review of utilization of MI within musculoskeletal health showed no studies contained children. More recently, the pediatric literature has started to focus on use of MI for chronic health conditions such as diabetes (Stanger et al., 2013), though studies reporting on this within pediatric chronic pain populations were not identified. Providers are advised to not underestimate the importance of eliciting feedback in order to ensure a shared understanding with patients and families around intent to engage in treatment and to resolve ambivalence regarding pursuing a recommended treatment.

The foundation for understanding MI requires an appreciation of the transtheoretical model of behavioral change (McConnaughy, Prochaska, & Velicer, 1983; Prochaska & DiClemente, 1984), also referred to as stages of change (McConnaughy, DiClemente, Prochaska, & Velicer, 1989; McConnaughy et al., 1983) or readiness to change (Prochaska, Norcross, & DiClemente, 1994). This model posits multiple progressive "stages" (including precontemplation, contemplation, preparation, action, and maintenance) that are associated with specific thoughts and behaviors that best characterize each stage. Critical to the success of a particular treatment recommendation is the "match" of the desired strategy or recommendation to the patient's current stage. Smoking cessation, weight loss, and chronic pain disorders have all been targets of change using this model (Prochaska & DiClemente, 1983; Snow et al., 1993). Assessing readiness to adopt a self-management approach to chronic pain led to the development of the Pain Stages of Change Questionnaire (Kerns, Rosenberg, Jamison, Caudill, & Haythornthwaite, 1997), which was originally validated in adult chronic pain samples and has more recently been validated using parallel forms developed for use with adolescents with chronic pain and their parents (Guite, Logan, Simons, Blood, & Kerns, 2011).

The Nuts and Bolts of CBT for Treatment of Chronic Pain

Before delving into the CBT model's treatment of chronic pain, it will be important to set the stage early in treatment. Providing education to the patient about their symptoms through use of metaphor/analogies is emphasized along with behavioral components of sleep and activity. The education that the patient receives provides rationale for learning and applying relaxation strategies as well as cognitive restructuring strategies.

Role of Psychoeducation

Psychoeducation is a key component of CBT and is even more important when working with a child, adolescent, or adult with chronic pain. A child, adolescent, or adult will often not understand the meaning of chronic pain. Thus, it will be helpful to define what chronic pain is for the patient and differentiate this type of pain from acute pain. Including examples will assist the patient in understanding what is going on in their body and what they can do about it. For example, one could describe touching a hot stove or accidentally slicing a finger with a sharp knife. Both can create injuries classified as acute pain, which serves a protective function by alerting the individual to take action (i.e., get away from the noxious situation, seek medical attention). In contrast, chronic pain is when an individual exhibits pain that typically lasts for longer than 3 months and after the body is no longer in immediate or im-minent danger. Our first inclination is to do the actions we would do if we touch a hot stove or cut ourselves with a sharp knife (e.g., rest, ice), but we now know that the same interventions we do for acute pain are not helpful for chronic pain. Further elaborating on the relation between stress, pain, anxiety, and depression will help the patient understand the interconnectedness of pain and emotions. Ensuring psycho-education is developmentally appropriate is important. The use of metaphor is a key ingredient to providing psychoeducation to the patient with chronic pain and can be a highly effective way to facilitate understanding of the problem across development (Coakley & Schechter, 2013). This is especially important because of the unseen na-ture of chronic pain, as such pain looks different than acute pain and is often invisible to other providers and people in the patient's life.

Coakley and Schechter (2013) provide some useful analogies to provide patients so that they can better understand what chronic pain is and how treatment can be helpful. To explain the persistence of pain despite the lack of imminent or immediate threat to the body, it can be helpful to introduce one of a variety of alarm metaphors. For example, the clinician can tell the patient that chronic pain is like an overactive car alarm. When the car gets gently bumped, the alarm goes off even when there is no sign of danger. Similar to cars with more sensitive alarms, people with more sensitive nervous systems have more false alarms (pain). Thus, the rationale for psy-chological intervention is the benefit of "retraining" the brain to reperceive the ex-perience of pain, and the skills and strategies learned through CBT can be helpful. Other analogies for the alarm include a haywire doorbell and broken alarm clock. By using metaphor and analogy, the clinician builds trust with a patient and creates a greater likelihood that the patient will follow-through with recommendations re-garding treatment.

▌The Gate Control Theory of Pain

Explaining the gate control theory of pain (Melzack & Wall, 1965; Palermo, 2012) to the patient with chronic pain is imperative, as it sets the stage for learning coping strategies to manage pain. It is important to explain that pain signals travel from the injury site up the spinal cord to the brain. The clinician can relay the importance of the brain's role of sending signals back to the spinal cord, which modulates (increases or decreases) pain. This is where psychological processes can come into play as pro-cesses such as what we think and how we feel can modulate the experience of pain (in addition to medication). Learning coping strategies can help to retrain the brain to reperceive how pain is experienced and help to calm down the sympathetic nervous system's fight-or-flight response. Oftentimes, individuals who play sports may play an entire game with a significant injury and experience little to no pain, only to real-ize after the game that they sustained a major injury. Eliciting from the patient why they just noticed this after the game will be helpful in having the patient understand the impact that thoughts ("I need to win the game") and feelings (adrenaline, eupho-ria) can have on the pain system. In the case of this individual's pain system, his/her thoughts and feelings during the game contributed to their dampened pain response and their ability to play through a significant injury.

Importance of Sleep

There is some evidence that sleep disturbance can increase sensitivity to pain (Lautenbacher, Kundermann, & Krieg, 2006) and that children and adolescents with persistent pain tend to have impaired sleep (Valrie, Bromberg, Palermo, & Schanberg, 2013). Sleep disturbance is a common issue for children and adolescents with chronic pain as there is a bidirectional relationship between pain and sleep. Pain can interfere with quality and quantity of sleep and insufficient sleep can interfere with pain coping during the day. Adequate sleep promotes tissue repair and psychological processes helpful for healing. According to the Centers for Disease Control and Prevention (2017), the recommended number of hours of sleep for school-age children (6-12 years) is 9 to 12 hours, 8 to 10 hours for 13- to 18-year-olds, and 7 or more hours per night for 18- to 60-year-old adults. Having persistent pain is associated with heightened physiological arousal and hypervigilance, which can make going to sleep difficult. Widespread pain is also associated with sleep difficulties in older adults (Chen, Hayman, Shmerling, Bean, & Leveille, 2011), and the relationship between chronic widespread pain and insomnia is reciprocal and both conditions tend to increase with age (McBeth, Wilkie, Bedson, Chew-Graham, & Lacey, 2015). Depressive symptoms in those with chronic pain predict severity of sleep disturbances (Lewin & Dahl, 1999; Palermo, 2012). Thus, it will be important early in treatment to establish whether the patient is obtaining the correct amount of sleep and ensure through psychoeducation that they understand the importance of completing this task.

Young and Kemper (2013) found that over one-third of their pediatric sample receiving care in an integrative clinic for chronic pain had sleep problems and that over half of caregivers requested additional counseling pertaining to sleep. In order to facilitate sleep, it will be helpful to complete a current assessment of a patient's sleep. This can include the schedule of sleep (what time the patient goes to bed/falls asleep, differences between workdays/schooldays and the weekend), whether there are phones/televisions in the bedroom, whether there is worry/sadness about loss of sleep, what occurs when there is awakening during the night, and how does the loss of sleep impact the individual during the day (Palermo, 2012). If the patient is endorsing inconsistency with their sleep schedule, using a cell phone or other electronic device prior to sleep, delayed onset/frequent awakenings at night, and loss of sleep, the clinician should work toward optimizing this important domain. Optimizing sleep means placing greater emphasis on sleep hygiene or keeping a consistent sleep schedule, limiting naps, ensuring the bedroom is only for sleeping (not studying or completing other activities), creating a relaxing routine before bed, and ensuring that electronics are not being used before bed or, better yet, are not present in the bedroom (Palermo, 2012).

Behavioral Activation and Physical Activity

As mentioned earlier, although the inclination of many patients with chronic pain is to rest and decrease activity, it is actually recommended that these individuals engage in some kind of physical activity. In CBT, this component of treatment is called behavioral activation. The key part of behavioral activation is scheduling activities to improve mood. Working with a physical therapist can help to improve functional abilities and address deconditioning or lack of range of motion for patients with chronic pain. It has been shown that physical activity such as exercise elevates mood and, in addition, increases an individual's pain threshold. For example, in the adult literature, a 2005 review of use of exercise for chronic low back pain in adults found that stretching and strengthening may improve pain and function (Hayden, Van Tulder, & Tomlinson, 2005). A 2017 systematic review of physical activity and exercise for chronic pain in adults found that exercise can reduce pain intensity, improve physical function, and increase quality of life (Geneen et al., 2017). Relatively less research has focused on exercise and physical activity among pediatric chronic pain samples until more recently (Kashikar-Zuck et al., 2010, 2013; Kashikar-Zuck, Myer, & Ting, 2012). Emerging evidence suggests that altered biomechanics may exist for youth with chronic widespread pain/juvenile fibromyalgia (JFM) (Sil et al., 2015). Initial intervention development efforts suggest efficacy for a combined CBT and neuromuscular retraining group treatment for adolescents with JFM holds promise for decreasing pain intensity and functional disability (Kashikar-Zuck, Tran, et al., 2016; Tran et al., 2017).

> ▶ **KEY POINT**
>
> The clinician's role in advocating for exercise and giving the rationale for such exercise is important. Just as acute pain can best be treated using rest, movement and exercise (often graded in nature) are indicated for those with chronic pain. A clinician can help a patient adhere to the treatment plan of exercise, with emphasis on pacing or not underdoing or overdoing activity.

Relaxation Strategies

Relaxation strategies are commonly introduced to individuals experiencing chronic pain and are also common to CBT. It is necessary to provide emphasis on stressing the importance of not just learning these strategies but applying them in the moment. Just like one can learn how to shoot a free throw in basketball, committing to the practice enables an individual to score at crucial points during the game. Although a patient may learn many different strategies and put them in their toolbox, some tools may work, some may not be as effective. The clinician will need to make the patient aware of connections between stress, muscle tension, and pain and how relaxation strategies can be helpful (Palermo, 2012). CBT and associated relaxation strategies have been found beneficial for physical functioning, improved pain, and improved quality of life for adults experiencing chronic pain (Abbott et al., 2017; Adachi, Fujino, Nakae, Mashimo, & Sasaki, 2014; Bernardy et al., 2013; Theadom, Cropley, Smith, Feigin, & McPherson, 2015; Williams et al., 2012). CBT and relaxation strategies have also been found to be beneficial for children experiencing chronic pain and can specifically reduce the intensity of pain in chronic headache, recurrent abdominal pain, fibromyalgia, and sickle cell disease (Eccleston et al., 2014). Relaxation strategies such as deep breathing, imagery, and progressive muscle relaxation (PMR) will be described later. The following section will discuss cognitive restructuring strategies.

Deep breathing, also called diaphragmatic breathing or belly breathing, is one type of strategy that can be taught to a patient with chronic pain to assist with relaxation. Patients are instructed to place one hand on stomach and one hand on the chest as they breathe in through their nose for a count of five and then exhaling through the mouth slowly. They are instructed to notice that on inhalation the stomach moves out like a balloon, whereas during the exhalation, the stomach flattens like a pancake. The clinician can demonstrate this to the patient while lying on the floor and putting an object on the stomach to demonstrate what occurs during an inhalation and what occurs during an exhalation. For younger children, it may be helpful incorporating other objects such as balloons or bubbles to help. There are also multiple mobile apps that are readily available to facilitate this practice and encourage use outside of scheduled appointment sessions (Smith et al., 2015).

Imagery is another coping skill that allows the patient to create pleasant, relaxing, and calm images that allow for defocusing from pain. Brainstorming about what pleasant images a person finds calming and joyous is an important part of this exercise. The clinician can also go over with the patient in addition to incorporating their five senses. This exercise allows a patient to imagine "going" to another place in order to focus their attention away from their pain experience. This experience is ideally relaxing for the patient.

PMR was created by Edmund Jacobsen in the 1930s and was originally used with adults (Jacobsen, 1938). PMR teaches a patient to notice the difference in tense versus relaxed muscles by going through several different muscle groups. Generally speaking, muscles are held in tension for 5 to 7 seconds and then relaxed for 20 to 30 seconds. Muscle groups include the hand/wrist, arm/biceps, shoulders/neck, head, back, chest, stomach, and legs. It is imperative that the clinician takes into account the age of the patient, as younger patients will require more concrete and age-appropriate directions than older participants (Palermo, 2012).

Hypnosis (or hypnotherapy) is a self-regulation strategy that has been used with both children and adults with chronic pain. Abbott et al.'s (2017) systematic review of psychological interventions for recurrent pediatric abdominal pain found that hypnotherapy reduces pain intensity and pain frequency and may have long-term benefits according to one study. Adachi et al.'s (2014) meta-analysis of hypnosis for adult chronic pain found that this intervention is moderately effective compared with standard of care, with no differences in efficacy between hypnosis and other interventions. Hypnosis involves three parts: induction, deepening, and suggestions. A hypnotic trance is created to facilitate a state of relaxation, followed by the clinician making suggestions to change symptoms to decrease pain. Although hypnosis is a readily teachable and effective strategy for a wide range of painful problems (e.g., irritable bowel syndrome; Webb, Kukuruzovic, Catto-Smith, & Sawyer, 2007, needle-related pain; Birnie et al., 2014), it is recommended that clinicians receive supplemental or specialized training to use it most effectively (Palermo, 2012).

Biofeedback is a technique with broad application for various health-related concerns (Schwartz & Andrasik, 2003), including chronic pain disorders. It has considerable empirical support as a nonpharmacologic treatment for chronic pain in both pediatric (Eccleston et al., 2014; Powers et al., 2001; Scharff, Marcus, & Masek, 2002) and adult (Gereau et al., 2014; Peek, 2003) samples. Fundamentally, biofeedback utilizes external information captured about the body or body physiology that is shared with the patient to then self-modify their body state. Biofeedback generally utilizes electronic equipment in order to provide real-time physiologic feedback to the patient, most typically information about the patient's sympathetic and parasympathetic nervous system. Patients using this strategy are able to see their heart rate, muscle tension, and temperature; and the patient is able to change these physiologic processes through use of various relaxation strategies. Although biofeedback devices are becoming widely available, it is recommended that clinicians who wish to specialize in this treatment modality receive supplemental or specialized training to use it most effectively (Palermo, 2012).

Cognitive Restructuring and Emotion Regulation

Similarly to relaxation strategies, there is a broad base of support for cognitive restructuring as a component of CBT (Eccleston et al., 2014). An individual's thoughts and feelings may contribute to and exacerbate their experience with pain. Anxiety, depression, worry, pain catastrophizing (pain-related anxiety), kinesiophobia (fear of movement), and hyper-focusing on the pain are common experiences when having chronic pain. Challenging negative thoughts and modifying them with positive coping statements is a staple CBT intervention. Recognizing the intersection and relation between thoughts, feelings, behaviors, and physical sensations is a key component to CBT and is often completed with the help of a tracking diary referred to as a thought record. Helping the patient understand the rationality and helpfulness of thoughts and how they affect feelings, behaviors, and physical sensations is imperative. This type of treatment often entails treating thoughts as just thoughts that are not necessarily part of reality. Having the patient ask himself/herself, "what I am I worried about?", "what has happened when I thought this thought or worry before?", "what are the facts?", what else could happen?", and "how likely is this to happen?" can help the patient create more awareness of the thought they are having and if it is irrational/unhelpful (Rapee, Wignall, Spence, Lyneham, & Cobham, 2008). Helping a patient find the evidence for and against a certain thought can assist them in thinking more realistically about their experience, which can help with increasing function and decreasing their emotional reactiveness to pain. Through using relaxation strategies, and thinking about pain differently, the patient has an opportunity to better regulate their emotional experience, which can assist with "turning down" their pain system alarm in addition to their sympathetic nervous system.

Home Practice and SMART Goals

Home practice is an essential component to applying learned skills during therapy. It is important in the beginning of treatment to emphasize that although it is great to learn relaxation skills and thinking skills during contact with a provider/therapist, if these techniques are not practiced consistently, it will be more difficult to apply them when those skills are truly needed. One can use the analogy of muscle memory with running a marathon: if you do not practice running, it will be nearly impossible to run a marathon on the day you want to complete this task. When working with children, ensuring involvement of the parents in reinforcing practice will be important.

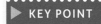

KEY POINT

Clinicians would be wise to incorporate specific, measurable, achievable, realistic/relevant, and timed (i.e., "SMART") goals into treatment plans that are specific, measurable, attainable, realistic, and time-limited (Bovend'Eerdt, Botell, & Wade, 2009).

The process of creating and discussing the SMART goals by a provider with a patient and parent/caregiver may also aid in the success of attaining desired outcomes and adherence to treatment recommendations (Fisher, Bromberg, Tai, & Palermo, 2016; Fisher & Palermo, 2016; Thompson, Broadbent, Bertino, & Staiger, 2016).

Parent-Management Strategies/Spousal Strategies

Parents of children with chronic pain play a pivotal role during treatment. Oftentimes, parents may have certain expectations for treatment (e.g., finding a cure), which may be at odds with difficult behavioral changes being asked (e.g., increased activity). When children have higher emotional distress from pain, maladaptive parental responses such as increased focus on pain, discounting the pain, and giving special privileges were associated with increased functional disability and somatic symptoms (Claar, Simons, & Logan, 2008). Lewandowski, Palermo, Stinson, Handley, and Chambers' (2010) systematic review found that poor family functioning is related more to pain-related disability rather than pain intensity. Thus, parents have a significant role to play in their child's treatment of chronic pain and interventions targeting parents is helpful. Palermo (2012) elaborates on several strategies for parents to use that reinforce function. These strategies include encouraging normal activity during pain episodes, eliminating status checks, praising a child's use of coping skills, and reducing behaviors that give attention to illness behaviors. More recent advances in family-focused interventions for youth with chronic pain have specifically targeted parents' own experience of distress and caregiving burden and show promise for parents of youth treated in an outpatient context (Guite et al., 2018).

There has been limited research with regard to spousal interventions for adults with chronic pain. Martire, Schulz, Helgeson, Small, and Saghafi's (2010) review of 33 studies and a subset of 25 meta-analyses for couples-based interventions for chronic physical illness showed that such interventions had significant effects on depression, marital functioning, and pain for patients with cardiovascular disease, chronic pain, human immunodeficiency virus, and type 2 diabetes. A recent randomized controlled trial of spouse-assisted training in pain coping skills for chronic low back pain showed that incorporation of a spouse during the multidisciplinary team intervention compared to standard multidisciplinary pain management or standard medical care led to less rumination about the pain (Abbasi et al., 2012). Specific interventions included providing education about chronic low back pain and cognitive-behavioral pain coping skills.

Family/Clinician Resources

When treating chronic pain, it is important that the patient, whether they are an adult or adolescent, has as much information as possible regarding what chronic pain is and how it can be treated. It is also important that providers in the community know what chronic pain is and how it can be treated. To this end, we typically recommend that parents of children read more about the condition through excellent resources such as Rachael Coakley's *When Your Child Hurts* (Coakley, 2016), and providers in the community who collaborate in the care of youth with chronic pain to become familiar with the problem through texts such as Tonya Palermo's *Cognitive-Behavioral*

Therapy for Chronic Pain in Children and Adolescents (Palermo, 2012). Technology through phone applications can also be used to improve engagement of children and adolescents in treatment. A 2015 published review (Smith et al., 2015) of Apple apps identified various phone applications for breathing (e.g., Breathe2Relax, Pranayama Free), general information (e.g., Simply Being—Guided Meditation for Relaxation), CBT (e.g., CBT4Kids Toolbox, CBT Tools for Kids), and sleep (e.g., Sleep Well!, iSleep Easy—Meditations for Restful Sleep) that can be beneficial for coping across the developmental life span.

█ Conclusion

Engel's biopsychosocial model (Engel, 1977) and its clinical application (Engel, 1980) illustrate the impact of cognitions, emotions, and the environment on one's experience with pain. This concept becomes ever more important when discussing strategies to manage chronic pain from a nonpharmacologic standpoint. Pain is not only a physical sensation but is a way in which an individual interprets, "apprehension of threat to their bodily or existential integrity" (Cohen et al., 2018). Thus, it is also amenable to interventions that impact these factors. There is substantial support for psychological strategies to treat chronic pain, including CBT and related strategies, as part of an interdisciplinary treatment plan. However, before treating chronic pain with CBT, clinicians and practitioners should make sure to consider how to best engage the patient in the desired treatment and outcome. Drawing on knowledge of the importance of the therapeutic alliance, MI, and understanding the patient's perception of pain and psychotherapy are essential considerations. These factors will assist the clinician to ensure that the intended referral is understood, agreed to, and ultimately implemented by the patient who must take ownership of engaging in the process. Once a patient is referred for treatment, it is imperative that the clinician maintains expectations for engagement and provides consistent messages about what chronic pain is and the interconnectedness between our thoughts, emotions (anxiety, depression), stress, and pain. Relaxation strategies to assist patients in managing their pain include deep breathing, imagery, PMR, hypnosis, and biofeedback. Improving sleep and increasing physical activity through pacing are also important. These strategies along with cognitive restructuring can help the patient to be more proactive as they face chronic pain and help to "turn down" their pain system's alarm and ultimately achieve confidence and satisfaction around their ability to effectively self-manage chronic pain.

REFERENCES

Abbasi, M., Dehghani, M., Keefe, F. J., Jafari, H., Behtash, H., & Shams, J. (2012). Spouse-assisted training in pain coping skills and the outcome of multidisciplinary pain management for chronic low back pain treatment: A 1-year randomized controlled trial. *European Journal of Pain, 16*(7), 1033–1043. doi:10.1002/j.1532-2149.2011.00097.x

Abbott, R. A., Martin, A. E., Newlove-Delgado, T. V., Bethel, A., Thompson-Coon, J., Whear, R., & Logan, S. (2017). Psychosocial interventions for recurrent abdominal pain in childhood. *The Cochrane Library, 1*, CD010971.

Adachi, T., Fujino, H., Nakae, A., Mashimo, T., & Sasaki, J. (2014). A meta-analysis of hypnosis for chronic pain problems: A comparison between hypnosis, standard care, and other psychological interventions. *International Journal of Clinical and Experimental Hypnosis, 62*(1), 1–28. doi:10.1080/00207144.2013.841471

Alperstein, D., & Sharpe, L. (2016). The efficacy of motivational interviewing in adults with chronic pain: A meta-analysis and systematic review. *The Journal of Pain, 17*(4), 393–403. doi:10.1016/j.jpain.2015.10.021

Anagnostis, C., Gatchel, R. J., & Mayer, T. G. (2004). The pain disability questionnaire: A new psychometrically sound measure for chronic musculoskeletal disorders. *Spine, 29*(20), 2290–2302.

Beck, A. T. (1963). Thinking and depression. *Archives of General Psychiatry, 9,* 324–333.

Beck, A. T., Rush, A. J., Shaw, B. F., & Emery, G. (1979). *Cognitive therapy of depression.* New York, NY: Guilford Press.

Beck, J. S. (2011). *Cognitive behavior therapy: Basics and beyond.* New York, NY: Guilford Press.

Beidas, R. S., Stewart, R. E., Walsh, L., Lucas, S., Downey, M. M., Jackson, K., . . . Mandell, D. S. (2015). Free, brief, and validated: Standardized instruments for low-resource mental health settings. *Cognitive and Behavioral Practice, 22*(1), 5–19. doi:10.1016/j.cbpra.2014.02.002

Bernardy, K., Klose, P., Busch, A. J., Choy, E. H. S., & Häuser, W. (2013). Cognitive behavioural therapies for fibromyalgia. *Cochrane Database of Systematic Reviews* (9). doi:10.1002/14651858.CD009796.pub2

Birnie, K. A., Noel, M., Parker, J. A., Chambers, C. T., Uman, L. S., Kisely, S. R., & McGrath, P. J. (2014). Systematic review and meta-analysis of distraction and hypnosis for needle-related pain and distress in children and adolescents. *Journal of Pediatric Psychology, 39*(8), 783–808. doi:10.1093/jpepsy/jsu029

Bovend'Eerdt, T. J. H., Botell, R. E., & Wade, D. T. (2009). Writing SMART rehabilitation goals and achieving goal attainment scaling: A practical guide. *Clinical Rehabilitation, 23*(4), 352–361. doi:10.1177/0269215508101741

Bursch, B., Walco, G. A., & Zeltzer, L. K. (1998). Clinical assessment and management of chronic pain and pain-associated disability syndrome. *Journal of Developmental and Behavioral Pediatrics, 19*(1), 45–53.

Cella, D., Yount, S., Rothrock, N., Gershon, R., Cook, K., Reeve, B., . . . Rose, M. (2007). The patient-reported outcomes measurement information system (PROMIS): Progress of an NIH Roadmap Cooperative Group during its first two years. *Medical Care, 45*(5 Suppl. 1), S3–S11. doi:10.1097/01.mlr.0000258615.42478.55

Centers for Disease Control and Prevention. (2017). *How much sleep do I need?* Retrieved from https://www.cdc.gov/sleep/about_sleep/how_much_sleep.html

Chen, Q., Hayman, L. L., Shmerling, R. H., Bean, J. F., & Leveille, S. G. (2011). Characteristics of chronic pain associated with sleep difficulty in older adults: The Maintenance of Balance, Independent Living, Intellect, and Zest in the Elderly (MOBILIZE) Boston Study. *Journal of the American Geriatrics Society, 59*(8), 1385–1392. doi:10.1111/j.1532-5415.2011.03544.x

Chilton, R., Pires-Yfantouda, R., & Wylie, M. (2012). A systematic review of motivational interviewing within musculoskeletal health. *Psychology, Health & Medicine, 17*(4), 392–407. doi:10.1080/13548506.2011.635661

Claar, R. L., Simons, L. E., & Logan, D. E. (2008). Parental response to children's pain: The moderating impact of children's emotional distress on symptoms and disability. *Pain, 138,* 172–179.

Coakley, R. M. (2016). *When your child hurts: Effective strategies to increase comfort, reduce stress, and break the cycle of chronic pain.* New Haven, CT: Yale University Press.

Coakley, R. M., & Schechter, N. L. (2013). Chronic pain is like . . . The clinical use of analogy and metaphor in the treatment of chronic pain in children. *Pediatric Pain Letter, 15*(1), 1–8.

Cohen, M., Quintner, J., & van Rysewyk, S. (2018). Reconsidering the International Association for the Study of Pain definition of pain. *PAIN Reports, 3*(2), e634. doi:10.1097/pr9.0000000000000634

Collier, R. (2018). "Complainers, malingerers and drug-seekers"—The stigma of living with chronic pain. *Canadian Medical Association Journal, 190*(7), E204.

Dworkin, R. H., Turk, D. C., Farrar, J. T., Haythornthwaite, J. A., Jensen, M. P., Katz, N. P., . . . Witter, J. (2005). Core outcome measures for chronic pain clinical trials: IMMPACT recommendations. *Pain, 113*(1–2), 9–19.

Eccleston, C., Hearn, L., & Williams, A. C. D. C. (2015). Psychological therapies for the management of chronic neuropathic pain in adults. *Cochrane Database of Systematic Reviews* (10). doi:10.1002/14651858.CD011259.pub2

Eccleston, C., Palermo, T. M., Williams, A., Lewandowski Holley, A., Morley, S., Fisher, E., & Law, E. (2014). Psychological therapies for the management of chronic and recurrent pain in children and adolescents. *Cochrane Database of Systematic Reviews* (5). doi:10.1002/14651858.CD003968.pub4

Engel, G. L. (1977). The need for a new medical model: A challenge for biomedicine. *Science, 196*, 129–136.

Engel, G. L. (1980). The clinical application of the biopsychosocial model. *American Journal of Psychiatry, 137*, 535–544.

Felitti, V. J., Anda, R. F., Nordenberg, D., Williamson, D. F., Spitz, A. M., Edwards, V., . . . Marks, J. S. (1998). Relationship of childhood abuse and household dysfunction to many of the leading causes of death in adults: The Adverse Childhood Experiences (ACE) Study. *American Journal of Preventive Medicine, 14*(4), 245–258. doi:10.1016/S0749-3797(98)00017-8

Fisher, E., Bromberg, M. H., Tai, G., & Palermo, T. M. (2016). Adolescent and parent treatment goals in an internet-delivered chronic pain self-management program: Does agreement of treatment goals matter? *Journal of Pediatric Psychology, 42*(6), 657–666. doi:10.1093/jpepsy/jsw098

Fisher, E., Heathcote, L., Palermo, T. M., de C Williams, A. C., Lau, J., & Eccleston, C. (2014). Systematic review and meta-analysis of psychological therapies for children with chronic pain. *Journal of Pediatric Psychology, 39*(8), 763–782. doi:10.1093/jpepsy/jsu008

Fisher, E., & Palermo, T. M. (2016). Goal pursuit in youth with chronic pain. *Children (Basel), 3*(4). doi:10.3390/children3040036

Gatchel, R. J. (2004). Comorbidity of chronic pain and mental health disorders: The biopsychosocial perspective. *American Psychologist, 59*(8), 795–805. doi:10.1037/0003-066X.59.8.795

Geneen, L. J., Moore, R. A., Clarke, C., Martin, D., Colvin, L. A., & Smith, B. H. (2017). Physical activity and exercise for chronic pain in adults: An overview of Cochrane Reviews. *The Cochrane Database of Systematic Reviews* (4), CD011279. doi:10.1002/14651858.CD011279.pub3

Gereau, R. W. IV., Sluka, K. A., Maixner, W., Savage, S. R., Price, T. J., Murinson, B. B., . . . Fillingim, R. B. (2014). A pain research agenda for the 21st century. *The Journal of Pain, 15*(12), 1203–1214. doi:10.1016/j.jpain.2014.09.004

Guite, J. W., Kim, S., Chen, C.-P., Sherker, J. L., Sherry, D. D., Rose, J. B., & Hwang, W.-T. (2014). Treatment expectations among adolescents with chronic musculoskeletal pain and their parents before an initial pain clinic evaluation. *The Clinical Journal of Pain, 30*(1), 17–26. doi:10.1097/AJP.0b013e3182851735

Guite, J. W., Logan, D. E., Ely, E. A., & Weisman, S. J. (2012). The ripple effect: Systems-level interventions to ameliorate pediatric pain. *Pain Management, 2*(6), 593–601. doi:10.2217/pmt.12.63

Guite, J. W., Logan, D. E., Simons, L. E., Blood, E. A., & Kerns, R. D. (2011). Readiness to change in pediatric chronic pain: Initial validation of adolescent and parent versions of the Pain Stages of Change Questionnaire. *Pain, 152*(10), 2301–2311.

Guite, J. W., Russell, B. S., Pantaleao, A., Thompson-Heller, A., Donohue, E., Galica, V., . . . Ohannessian, C. M. (2018). Parents as coping coaches for adolescents with chronic pain: A single-arm pilot feasibility trial of a brief, group-based, cognitive-behavioral intervention promoting caregiver self-regulation. *Clinical Practice in Pediatric Psychology, 6*(3), 223–237. doi:10.1037/cpp0000244

Hayden, J. A., Van Tulder, M. W., & Tomlinson, G. (2005). Systematic review: Strategies for using exercise therapy to improve outcomes in chronic low back pain. *Annals of Internal Medicine, 142*(9), 776–785.

Hayes, S. C., Pistorello, J., & Levin, M. E. (2012). Acceptance and commitment therapy as a unified model of behavior change. *The Counseling Psychologist, 40*(7), 976–1002. doi:10.1177/0011000012460836

Hayes, S. C., Strosahl, K. D., & Wilson, K. G. (1999). *Acceptance and commitment therapy: An experiential approach to behavior change.* New York, NY: Guilford Press.

Horvath, A. O., Del Re, A. C., Flückiger, C., & Symonds, D. (2011). Alliance in individual psychotherapy. *Psychotherapy, 48*(1), 9–16. doi:10.1037/a0022186

Hughes, L. S., Clark, J., Colclough, J. A., Dale, E., & McMillan, D. (2017). Acceptance and commitment therapy (ACT) for chronic pain: A systematic review and meta-analyses. *The Clinical Journal of Pain, 33*(6), 552–568. doi:10.1097/AJP.0000000000000425

Jacobsen, E. (1938). *Progressive relaxation.* Chicago, IL: University of Chicago Press.

Jordan, A. L., Eccleston, C., & Osborn, M. (2007). Being a parent of the adolescent with complex chronic pain: An interpretative phenomenological analysis. *European Journal of Pain, 11*, 49–56.

Kashikar-Zuck, S., Carle, A., Barnett, K., Goldschneider, K. R., Sherry, D. D., Mara, C. A., . . . DeWitt, E. M. (2016). Longitudinal evaluation of Patient Reported Outcomes Measurement Information Systems (PROMIS) measures in pediatric chronic pain. *Pain, 157*(2), 339–347. doi:10.1097/j.pain.0000000000000378

Kashikar-Zuck, S., Flowers, S. R., Strotman, D., Sil, S., Ting, T. V., & Schikler, K. N. (2013). Physical activity monitoring in adolescents with juvenile fibromyalgia: Findings from a clinical trial of cognitive-behavioral therapy. *Arthritis Care & Research (Hoboken), 65*(3), 398–405. doi:10.1002/acr.21849

Kashikar-Zuck, S., Flowers, S. R., Verkamp, E., Ting, T. V., Lynch-Jordan, A. M., Graham, T. B., . . . Lovell, D. (2010). Actigraphy-based physical activity monitoring in adolescents with juvenile primary fibromyalgia syndrome. *Journal of Pain, 11*(9), 885–893. doi: 10.1016/j.jpain.2009.12.009

Kashikar-Zuck, S., Myer, G., & Ting, T. V. (2012). Can behavioral treatments be enhanced by integrative neuromuscular training in the treatment of juvenile fibromyalgia? *Pain Management, 2*(1), 9–12. doi:10.2217/pmt.11.60

Kashikar-Zuck, S., Tran, S. T., Barnett, K., Bromberg, M. H., Strotman, D., Sil, S., . . . Myer, G. D. (2016). A qualitative examination of a new combined cognitive-behavioral and neuromuscular training intervention for juvenile fibromyalgia. *The Clinical Journal of Pain, 32*(1), 70–81. doi:10.1097/AJP.0000000000000221

Kerns, R. D., Rosenberg, R., Jamison, R. N., Caudill, M. A., & Haythornthwaite, J. (1997). Readiness to adopt a self-management approach to chronic pain: The pain stages of change questionnaire (PSOCQ). *Pain, 72*(1–2), 227–234.

Lautenbacher, S., Kundermann, B., & Krieg, J.-C. (2006). Sleep deprivation and pain perception. *Sleep Medicine Reviews, 10*(5), 357–369.

Lewandowski, A. S., Palermo, T. M., Stinson, J., Handley, S., & Chambers, C. T. (2010). Systematic review of family functioning in families of children and adolescents with chronic pain. *The Journal of Pain, 11*(11), 1027–1038. doi:10.1016/j.jpain.2010.04.005

Lewin, D. S., & Dahl, R. E. (1999). Importance of sleep in the management of pediatric pain. *Journal of Developmental and Behavioral Pediatrics, 20*(4), 244–252. doi:10.1097/00004703-199908000-00006

Martire, L. M., Schulz, R., Helgeson, V. S., Small, B. J., & Saghafi, E. M. (2010). Review and meta-analysis of couple-oriented interventions for chronic illness. *Annals of Behavioral Medicine, 40*(3), 325–342. doi:10.1007/s12160-010-9216-2

McBeth, J., Wilkie, R., Bedson, J., Chew-Graham, C., & Lacey, R. J. (2015). Sleep disturbance and chronic widespread pain. *Current Rheumatology Reports, 17*(1), 469. doi:10.1007/s11926-014-0469-9

McConnaughy, E. A., DiClemente, C. C., Prochaska, J. O., & Velicer, W. F. (1989). Stages of change in psychotherapy: A follow-up report. *Psychotherapy: Theory, Research & Practice, 26*(4), 494–503.

McConnaughy, E. A., Prochaska, J. O., & Velicer, W. F. (1983). Stages of change in psychotherapy: Measurement and sample profiles. *Psychotherapy: Theory, Research & Practice, 20*(3), 368–375.

McCracken, L. M., & Iverson, G. L. (2002). Disrupted sleep patterns and daily functioning in patients with chronic pain. *Pain Research & Management, 7*(2), 75–79. doi:10.1155/2002/579425

McGrath, P. J., Walco, G. A., Turk, D., Dworkin, R. H., Brown, M. T., Davidson, K., . . . Zeltzer, L. (2008). Core outcome domains and measures for pediatric acute and chronic/recurrent pain clinical trials: PedIMMPACT recommendations. *The Journal of Pain, 9*(9), 771–783. doi:10.1016/j.jpain.2008.04.007

Melzack, R., & Wall, P. D. (1965). Pain mechanisms: A new theory. *Science, 150*(3699), 971–979.

Miller, W. R., & Rollnick, S. (2012). *Motivational interviewing: Helping people change.* New York, NY: Guilford Press.

Nelson, S., Simons, L. E., & Logan, D. (2018). The incidence of adverse childhood experiences (ACEs) and their association with pain-related and psychosocial impairment in youth with chronic pain. *The Clinical Journal of Pain, 34*(5), 402–408.

Palermo, T. M. (2012). *Cognitive-behavioral therapy for chronic pain in children and adolescents.* New York, NY: Oxford University Press.

Palermo, T. M., & Chambers, C. T. (2005). Parent and family factors in pediatric chronic pain and disability: An integrative approach. *Pain, 119,* 1–4.

Peek, C. J. (2003). A primer of biofeedback instrumentation. In M. S. Schwartz & F. Andrasik (Eds.), *Biofeedback: A practitioner's guide* (3rd ed., pp. 43–87). New York, NY: Guilford Press.

Powers, S. W., Mitchell, M. J., Byars, K. C., Bentti, A. L., LeCates, S. L., & Hershey, A. D. (2001). A pilot study of one-session biofeedback training in pediatric headache. *Neurology, 56*(1), 133.

Prochaska, J., Norcross, J., & DiClemente, C. (1994). *Changing for good: A revolutionary six-stage program for overcoming bad habits and moving your life positively forward.* New York, NY: William Morrow.

Prochaska, J. O., & DiClemente, C. C. (1983). Stages and processes of self-change of smoking: Toward an integrative model of change. *Journal of Consulting and Clinical Psychology, 51*(3), 390–395.

Prochaska, J. O., & DiClemente, C. C. (1984). *The transtheoretical approach; crossing traditional boundaries of therapy.* Homewood, IL: Dow Jones-Irwin.

Puzino, K., Guite, J. W., Moore, M., Lewen, M. O., & Williamson, A. A. (2017). The relationship between parental responses to pain, pain catastrophizing, and adolescent sleep in adolescents with chronic pain. *Children's Health Care*, 1–22. doi:10.1080/02739615.2017.1327358

Rapee, R., Wignall, A., Spence, S., Lyneham, H., & Cobham, V. (2008). *Helping your anxious child: A step-by-step guide for parents*. Oakland, CA: New Harbinger.

Rogers, C., & Farson, R. (1987). Active listening. In R. G. Newman, M. A. Danzinger, & M. Cohen (Eds.), *Communicating in business today*. Lexington, MA: D. C. Heath and Company.

Rogers, C. R. (1957). The necessary and sufficient conditions of therapeutic personality change. *Journal of Consulting Psychology, 21*(2), 95–103. doi:10.1037/h0045357

Sachs-Ericsson, N. J., Sheffler, J. L., Stanley, I. H., Piazza, J. R., & Preacher, K. J. (2017). When emotional pain becomes physical: Adverse childhood experiences, pain, and the role of mood and anxiety disorders. *Journal of Clinical Psychology, 73*(10), 1403–1428. doi:10.1002/jclp.22444

Salazar, A., Dueñas, M., Mico, J. A., Ojeda, B., Agüera-Ortiz, L., Cervilla, J. A., & Failde, I. (2013). Undiagnosed mood disorders and sleep disturbances in primary care patients with chronic musculoskeletal pain. *Pain Medicine, 14*(9), 1416–1425. doi:10.1111/pme.12165

Scharff, L., Marcus, D. A., & Masek, B. J. (2002). A controlled study of minimal-contact thermal biofeedback treatment in children with migraine. Journal of Pediatric Psychology, 27(2), 109-119.

Schwartz, M. S., & Andrasik, F. (Eds.). (2003). *Biofeedback: A practitioner's guide* (3rd ed.). New York, NY: Guilford Press.

Sil, S., Thomas, S., DiCesare, C., Strotman, D., Ting, T. V., Myer, G., & Kashikar-Zuck, S. (2015). Preliminary evidence of altered biomechanics in adolescents with juvenile fibromyalgia. *Arthritis Care & Research (Hoboken), 67*(1), 102–111. doi:10.1002/acr.22450

Smith, K., Iversen, C., Kossowsky, J., O'Dell, S., Gambhir, R., & Coakley, R. (2015). Apple apps for the management of pediatric pain and pain-related stress. *Clinical Practice in Pediatric Psychology, 3*(2), 93–107. doi:10.1037/cpp0000092

Snow, M. G., Kerns, R. D., Rosenberg, R., Jarvis, J. A., McCourt, M. S., & Prochaska, J. O. (1993). *Stages of change for chronic pain patients: Development of a questionnaire to assess readiness to change*. Paper presented at the Society of Behavioral Medicine, San Francisco, CA.

Stanger, C., Ryan, S. R., Delhey, L. M., Thrailkill, K., Li, Z., Li, Z., & Budney, A. J. (2013). A multicomponent motivational intervention to improve adherence among adolescents with poorly controlled type 1 diabetes: A pilot study. *Journal of Pediatric Psychology, 38*(6), 629–637. doi:10.1093/jpepsy/jst032

Strupp, H. H., & Binder, J. L. (1984). *Psychotherapy in a new key: A guide to time-limited dynamic psychotherapy*. New York, NY: Basic Books.

Sullivan, M. J. L., Bishop, S. R., & Pivik, J. (1995). The pain catastrophizing scale: Development and validation. *Psychological Assessment, 7*(4), 524–532. doi:10.1037/1040-3590.7.4.524

Sulmasy, L. S., López, A. M., & Horwitch, C. A., American College of Physicians Ethics, & Professionalism Human Rights Committee. (2017). Ethical implications of the electronic health record: In the service of the patient. *Journal of General Internal Medicine, 32*(8), 935–939.

Tegethoff, M., Belardi, A., Stalujanis, E., & Meinlschmidt, G. (2015). Comorbidity of mental disorders and chronic pain: Chronology of onset in adolescents of a national representative cohort. *The Journal of Pain, 16*(10), 1054–1064. doi:10.1016/j.jpain.2015.06.009

Theadom, A., Cropley, M., Smith, H. E., Feigin, V. L., & McPherson, K. (2015). Mind and body therapy for fibromyalgia. *Cochrane Database of Systematic Reviews* (4). doi:10.1002/14651858.CD001980.pub3

Thompson, E. L., Broadbent, J., Bertino, M. D., & Staiger, P. K. (2016). Do pain-related beliefs influence adherence to multidisciplinary rehabilitation? A systematic review. *The Clinical Journal of Pain, 32*(2), 164–178. doi:10.1097/AJP.0000000000000235

Tran, S. T., Guite, J. W., Pantaleao, A., Pfeiffer, M., Myer, G. D., Sil, S., . . . Kashikar-Zuck, S. (2017). Preliminary outcomes of a cross-site cognitive-behavioral and neuromuscular integrative training intervention for juvenile fibromyalgia. *Arthritis Care & Research, 69*(3), 413–420. doi:10.1002/acr.22946

Tunks, E. R., Crook, J., & Weir, R. (2008). Epidemiology of chronic pain with psychological comorbidity: Prevalence, risk, course, and prognosis. *The Canadian Journal of Psychiatry/ La Revue canadienne de psychiatrie, 53*(4), 224–234.

Turk, D. C., Dworkin, R. H., Burke, L. B., Gershon, R., Rothman, M., Scott, J., . . . Wyrwich, K. W. (2006). Developing patient-reported outcome measures for pain clinical trials: IMMPACT recommendations. *Pain, 125*(3), 208–215. doi:10.1016/j.pain.2006.09.028

Valrie, C. R., Bromberg, M. H., Palermo, T., & Schanberg, L. E. (2013). A systematic review of sleep in pediatric pain populations. *Journal of Developmental and Behavioral Pediatrics, 34*(2), 120–128. doi:10.1097/DBP.0b013e31827d5848

Walker, L. S., & Greene, J. W. (1991). The functional disability inventory: Measuring a neglected dimension of child health status. *Journal of Pediatric Psychology, 16*(1), 39–58. doi:10.1093/jpepsy/16.1.39

Webb, A. N., Kukuruzovic, R. H., Catto-Smith, A. G., & Sawyer, S. M. (2007). Hypnotherapy for treatment of irritable bowel syndrome. *Cochrane Database of Systematic Reviews* (4), CD005110.

Welmers-van de Poll, M. J., Roest, J. J., Stouwe, T., Akker, A. L., Stams, G. M., Escudero, V., & Swart, J. W. (2018). Alliance and treatment outcome in family-involved treatment for youth problems: A three-level meta-analysis. *Clinical Child and Family Psychology Review, 21*(2), 146–170. doi:10.1007/s10567-017-0249-y

Williams, A. C. D. C., Eccleston, C., & Morley, S. (2012). Psychological therapies for the management of chronic pain (excluding headache) in adults. *Cochrane Database of Systematic Reviews* (11). doi:10.1002/14651858.CD007407.pub3

Wolpe, J. (1973). *The practice of behavior therapy* (2nd ed.). Oxford, England: Pergamon.

World Health Organization. (2018). *World Health Organization Composite International Diagnostic Interview (CIDI) version 3.0—About the WHO WMH-CIDI.* Retrieved from https://www.hcp.med.harvard.edu/wmhcidi/about-the-who-wmh-cidi/

Young, L., & Kemper, K. J. (2013). Integrative care for pediatric patients with pain. *The Journal of Alternative and Complementary Medicine, 19*(7), 627–632. doi:10.1089/acm.2012.0368

CHAPTER 7

PHARMACOLOGIC MANAGEMENT OF PAIN

Trinh Pham

Pharmacologic Management of Pain

Pain can arise from a broad variety of causes and can be categorized according to duration (acute vs. chronic) or the underlying mechanisms causing the pain (nociceptive vs. neuropathic vs. inflammatory). Healthcare providers should be knowledgeable about the analgesic options that are available and the types of pain that may be responsive to those analgesics. There are three broad categories of analgesic medications—nonopioid analgesics, opioid analgesics, and adjuvant analgesics—that can be used to manage pain symptoms. A multimodal approach to pain management using a combination of these different categories of analgesics with different mechanisms of action may improve pain control via additive or synergistic effects of each of these categories of drugs in addition to reducing the risk of adverse effects because lower doses of each drug will be utilized. A sound understanding of the pharmacology of analgesic medications and their appropriate use facilitates effective prescribing, administration, and dispensing of the analgesics used to manage a patient's pain diagnosis. This chapter reviews the pharmacologic approach to the management of pain, the goal of which is to maximize efficacy of analgesic drug therapy while minimizing adverse effects and toxicities.

Nonopioid Analgesics

Nonopioid analgesics include acetaminophen and nonsteroidal anti-inflammatory drugs (NSAIDs). NSAIDs possess analgesic, anti-inflammatory, and anti-pyretic effects. Unlike NSAIDs, acetaminophen has no anti-inflammatory activity. These nonopioid analgesics are effective for the management of mild to moderate pain, and NSAIDs are effective for pain that has an inflammatory component.

▌Nonsteroidal Anti-inflammatory Drugs

NSAIDs are effective anti-inflammatory, antipyretic, and analgesic agents that are commonly used in the treatment of acute and chronic pain, rheumatoid arthritis, and osteoarthritis. They exert their pharmacologic effects via inhibition of one or both isoforms of the cyclooxygenase (COX) enzymes (COX-1 and COX-2), which catalyze the conversion of arachidonic acid to prostaglandins (PGs) and thromboxanes (Theken, 2018). Drugs that inhibit both COX-1 and COX-2 are known as nonselective NSAIDs (nsNSAIDs) and drugs that inhibit only COX-2 are referred to as selective NSAIDs. Inhibition of COX-1 is thought to be principally responsible for the adverse effects following prolonged administration of nonselective COX inhibitors, whereas selective COX-2 inhibition accounts for the anti-inflammatory, antipyretic, and analgesic efficacy of NSAIDs (Huntjens, Danhof, & Della Pasqua, 2005). COX-1 is constitutively expressed in most tissue types, and the PGs produced by this isoform mediate functions such as cytoprotection of the gastric mucosa, regulation of renal blood flow, and platelet aggregation. As a consequence, nsNSAIDs that inhibit not only COX-2 but also COX-1 lead to a greater risk of adverse effects such as gastrointestinal (GI) ulceration, bleeding, and nephrotoxicity. COX-2 is an inducible enzyme and its expression is highly restricted under basal conditions; however, its expression is greatly increased at inflammatory sites in response to cytokines such as interferon γ, tumor necrosis factor α, and interleukin 1 (Bacchi, Palumbo, Sponta, & Coppolino, 2012). PGE2 and PGI2 mediate central and peripheral nociceptive responses. Additionally, the decrease in the synthesis of PGE2 and PGI2, which are also considered to be vasodilating PGs, produces anti-inflammatory action and indirect reduction of edema. Thus, NSAIDs exert their analgesic effects by inhibiting PGs that promote peripheral and central sensitization (Bacchi et al., 2012), and they are effective in treating pain that occurs as a consequence of COX pathway activation, such as with acute injuries or arthritis (Theken, 2018).

All NSAIDs inhibit COX enzymes; however, there is marked diversity within the class with regard to their chemical properties, pharmacokinetics, and degree of selectivity for COX-2 over COX-1. NSAIDs may be classified on the basis of their in vitro COX enzyme selectivity (Table 7-1) (Bacchi et al., 2012; Warner et al., 1999) or their chemical structure (Table 7-2) (Antman et al., 2007; Wickham, 2017). Although COX selectivity characteristics of individual NSAIDs have been determined in vitro, it is difficult to translate the clinical risk of adverse effects for specific patients based on COX-2 selectivity. The differences in the NSAID characteristics may contribute to the variability in analgesic efficacy, adverse effect profile, and patient preferences for specific NSAIDs. Studies comparing the efficacy of individual NSAIDs have not identified greater efficacy of any individual NSAID over another; therefore, the analgesic efficacy of distinct NSAIDs is considered to be similar and no one drug is considered to be more effective than others within the class (Theken, 2018). The choice of a particular NSAID depends on the specific pharmacokinetic properties, adverse effect profile, availability, and cost of the individual agents. NSAIDs that are designed with enhanced dissolution and rapid absorption properties facilitate a shorter time to analgesic effect, which is a desirable characteristic for treating acute pain. NSAIDs with extended half-lives achieve stable drug concentrations with less frequent dosing

Table 7–1. Classification of NSAIDs Based on Their In Vitro COX-2 Inhibition Activity

Classification	Description	Drugs
Group 1 (<5-fold COX-2 selectivity)	Poorly selective NSAIDs that fully inhibit both COX-1 and COX-2	Aspirin, diclofenac, diflunisal, flurbiprofen, ibuprofen, indomethacin, ketoprofen, ketorolac, naproxen, piroxicam, sulindac, tolmetin
Group 2 (5- to 50-fold COX-2 selectivity)	NSAIDs capable of inhibiting both COX-1 and COX-2 with preferential selectivity toward COX-2	Celecoxib, etodolac, meloxicam
Group 3 (>50-fold COX-2 selectivity)	NSAIDs that strongly inhibit COX-2 but only weakly inhibit COX-1	Rofecoxib (no longer on the market in the United States)
Group 4	NSAIDs that seem to be only weak inhibitors of both COX-1 and COX-2	Sodium salicylate, nabumetone

COX, cyclooxygenase; NSAID, nonsteroidal anti-inflammatory drug.
Adapted from Bacchi, S., Palumbo, P., Sponta, A., & Coppolino, M. F. (2012). Clinical pharmacology of non-steroidal anti-inflammatory drugs: A review. *Anti-Inflammatory & Anti-Allergy Agents in Medicinal Chemistry, 11*, 52–64; Warner, T. D., Giuliano, F., Vojnovic, I., Bukasa, A., Mitchell, J. A., & Vane, J. R. (1999). Nonsteroidal rug selectivities for cyclo-oxygenase-1 rather than cyclo-oxygenase-2 are associated with human gastrointestinal toxicity: A full *in vitro* analysis. *Proceedings of the National Academy of Sciences, 96*, 7563–7568.

and are preferred for treating chronic, persistent pain, with an understanding that the risk of adverse effects is increased because of the long half-life. NSAIDs have an analgesic ceiling dose, above which only toxicity occurs with no additional pain relief. Because there is high interpatient variability in response to individual NSAIDs, it is clinically reasonable to switch to another drug member of the NSAID class if there is inadequate response after a minimum of 1 month therapy of a particular NSAID (Simon & Strand, 1997).

There are at least 20 different NSAID available in the United States, with formulations ranging from tablet, capsule, solution, suspension, suppository, injectable, and topical application (Table 7-2). In addition to oral formulations, acetaminophen and ibuprofen are available for parenteral administration. Diclofenac is available for topical application as a patch, gel, or solution. Aspirin, acetaminophen, and indomethacin are also formulated as suppositories. All NSAIDs are available by prescription with the exceptions of aspirin, ibuprofen, naproxen, and ketoprofen, which are also currently available over the counter (OTC) in the United States.

The availability of a topical NSAID formulation is beneficial because it reduces the likelihood of a patient experiencing adverse effects associated with systemic therapy. The topical NSAID is applied directly to the skin and it reaches only local tissue to achieve desired therapeutic effect with minimal systemic absorption (McPherson & Cimino, 2013). The most common adverse effect is local skin irritation or application site reaction, which includes dry skin, erythema, irritation, paresthesias, and pruritus. Although systemic adverse effects are less common with topical NSAIDs, patients have reported experiencing GI upset and headache (McPherson & Cimino, 2013). The topical NSAIDs available to treat painful conditions in the United States include diclofenac sodium 1% gel approved for relief of pain because of osteoarthritis

Table 7–2. Commonly Prescribed NSAIDs and Acetaminophen

Class/Drugs (Formulation)	Usual Dose (mg) (Max Dose in mg/d)	Half-life	Comments	Adverse Effects
Salicylic Acids				• **Gastrointestinal (BBW)**
Aspirin (acetylsalicylic acid) (PO, supp)	325–1,000 every 4–6 h (4,000)	0.25 h	OTC/Rx Irreversible inhibition of platelet aggregation	– Mild: nausea, heart burn, dyspepsia, abdominal pain, diarrhea in 20–40% of patients
				– Moderate: GI mucosal erosions and asymptomatic ulcers in 15–30% of patients; may heal spontaneously
Diflunisal (PO)	250–500 every 8–12 h (1,500)	8–13 h		– Severe: symptomatic ulcers, with/without bleeding, can be life threatening (1–2% of users; mortality 10%)
				• **Cardiovascular (BBW)**
Salsalate (PO)	1,500 twice daily (arthritis)	1 h		– MI, CVA, CHF, thrombosis, sudden cardiac death
				– Greater risk with COX-2 inhibitors
Nonacetylated Acids				• **Renal**
Choline magnesium trisalicylate (PO)	500–1,500 every 8–12 h (4,500)	2–3 h	Elderly: 750 every 8 h No effect on platelets	– Greatest risk during first 4–6 weeks
				– Acute kidney injury
Propionic Acid Derivatives				– Renal prostaglandins affect systemic vascular resistance and may lead to hypertension, sodium and water retention, edema, hyperkalemia, interstitial nephritis
Fenoprofen (PO)	200 every 4–6 h (3,200)	2–3 h		– **High risk:**
				– ibuprofen, ketoprofen, fenoprofen, indomethacin, piroxicam
Flurbiprofen (PO)	50–100 twice daily to three times a day (300)	5.7 h		– **Intermediate risk:** diclofenac, sulindac
				– **Low risk:** naproxen, nonaspirin salicylates
				• **Hypersensitivity Reactions**
				Lowest risk with COX-2 inhibitors
Ibuprofen (PO, IV)	PO: 200–400 every 4–6 h (1,200 OTC) (2,400 Rx) IV (RX only): 400–800 over 30 minutes every 6 h (3,200)	1.8–2.5 h	OTC/Rx Reversible inhibition of platelet aggregation	**Generalized** – Anaphylaxis, severe bronchospasms within minutes **Respiratory**
Ketoprofen (PO)	25–50 every 6–8 h (300)	2–4 h	OTC/Rx	– Acute: aspirin induced or exacerbated asthma
				– Delayed: pneumonitis
Naproxen (PO)	250 every 12 h (1,000)	12–17 h	Rx only	**Administer NSAIDs cautiously to elderly patients with already compromised renal function, heart failure, or hypertension**

(continued)

Table 7–2. Commonly Prescribed NSAIDs and Acetaminophen (*continued*)

Class/Drugs (Formulation)	Usual Dose (mg) (Max Dose in mg/d)	Half-life	Comments	Adverse Effects
Naproxen sodium (PO)	Acute pain: 550 every 12 h or 275 every 6–8 h (1,100)		OTC/Rx	
Indoles				
Indomethacin (PO and Supp)	25 twice daily to three times a day	4.5 h	High risk for CNS side effect	
Sulindac (PO)	150 twice daily	8–16.4 h		
Pyrrolacetic Acid				
Ketorolac (PO, IV/IM, nasal)	Parenteral: 30–60 IM or 30 IV initial dose; then 15–30 IV every 6 h PO: 10 every 4–6 h Nasal: One spray (15.75 mg) in each nostril every 6–8 h	4–7 h	Max 5 days May cause renal failure in elderly or hypovolemic patients	
Phenylacetic Acids				
Diclofenac potassium (PO)	Capsule: 25 four times a day Tablet: 50 three times a day (150)	1–2 h		
Diclofenac epolamine (patch)	Apply one patch twice daily to painful area	12 h	Apply only to intact skin	
Diclofenac sodium (gel, solution)	Gel and solution dosing is joint specific for osteoarthritis	79 h		

	Dose (mg)	Half-life	Notes	BBW
Indoleacetic Acid				
Etodolac	200–400 every 6 h (1,000)	6–7 h		
Oxicams				
Piroxicam (PO)	10–20 daily	30–80 h		
Meloxicam (PO)	7.5 daily (15)	16–24 h		
Anthranilic Acids				
Mefenamic acid (PO)	250 every 6 h (1,000)	2–3.3 h		
Meclofenamate (PO)	50–100 every 4–6 h (400)		Max 7 days	
Diaryl Heterocyclics (COX-2 Selective Inhibitor)				
Celecoxib (PO)	200 twice daily (400)	11 h	No antiplatelet effects Contraindicated in patients with sulfonamide allergy	
para-Aminophenol				
Acetaminophen (PO, IV, supp)	PO: 325–1,000 every 4–6 h (4,000) IV: 1,000 every 6 h (4,000) OTC max dose: 3,000 mg		OTC/Rx Parenteral formulation used for postoperative pain	• **Hepatotoxicity**

BBW, black box warning; CHF, congestive heart failure; CNS, central nervous system; COX, cyclooxygenase; CVA, cerebrovascular accident; GI, gastrointestinal; h, hour; IM, intramuscular; IV, intravenous; max, maximum; MI, myocardial infarction; OTC, over the counter; PO, by mouth; Rx, prescription; sup, suppository.

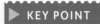

▶ KEY POINT

NSAIDs exert their pharmacologic effects via inhibition of one or both isoforms of the COX enzymes.

in joints such as the hands and knees that are amenable to topical treatment, diclofenac sodium topical solution 1.5% w/w in 45.5% dimethyl sulfoxide approved for osteoarthritis of the knees, and diclofenac epolamine 1.3% patch approved for topical treatment of acute pain because of minor strains, sprains, and contusions (Table 7-2) (McPherson & Cimino, 2013). The topical product should be administered directly to the desired site of action and it should be noted that the topical NSAIDs should not be used for hip osteoarthritis.

▌Adverse Effects of NSAIDs

Many potential adverse effects are associated with the use of NSAIDs, and there are differences in the adverse effect profile of COX-1 and COX-2 inhibitors. The inhibition of PGs leads to adverse effects that include GI complications, cardiovascular (CV) events, nephrotoxicity, exacerbation of hypertension, and fluid retention.

GI adverse effects

NSAIDs cause an increased risk of serious GI adverse effects such as gastric and duodenal ulcers because of systemic inhibition of PG synthesis, which results in a decrease in the protective barriers associated with gastric and duodenal mucosa. The GI side effects may be categorized as mild, moderate, or severe (Table 7-2) (Wickham, 2017). The risk factors for the development of GI-related side effects with NSAIDs include longer duration of NSAID usage, higher dosage, age over 60 years, past history of peptic ulcer disease, infection with *Helicobacter pylori*, alcohol use, combination therapy with corticosteroids, antiplatelet agents, anticoagulants, and/or selective serotonin inhibitors and patients who are frail (Bardou & Barkun, 2010; Meara & Simon, 2013). In order to prevent GI side effects from occurring, patients should use the lowest effective dose possible for the shortest duration of time to treat their pain. The addition of GI protective agents such as a proton pump inhibitor (PPI) like pantoprazole, omeprazole, or esomeprazole or an H2 antagonist like famotidine or ranitidine has been shown to decrease the incidence of gastric and duodenal ulcers (Dhillon, 2011; Goldstein et al., 2010; Laine et al., 2012), and guidelines from the American College of Gastroenterology recommend the use of once-daily PPI with a nsNSAID to decrease the incidence of NSAID-induced ulcers (Lanza, Chan, & Quigley, 2009). The COX-2 inhibitors have less potential to damage the GI mucosa than nsNSAIDs (Meara & Simon, 2013), and the risk of ulcer bleeding is comparable in patients with a history of peptic ulcer disease receiving a COX-2 inhibitor alone or a nsNSAID with a PPI (Chan et al., 2002). Primary prevention of NSAID-induced ulcers includes avoiding unnecessary use of NSAIDs, using acetaminophen or nonacetylated salicylates when possible, using the lowest effective dose of an NSAID, or switching to a selective COX-2 inhibitor in patients at high risk for NSAID-induced ulcers without CV risk. GI toxicity is greater with NSAIDs that have a long half-life (Table 7-2) and slow-release formulations. For prophylaxis or prevention of NSAID-induced ulcers, a PPI or misoprostol, a PGE1 analog, should be considered in patients with NSAID-induced ulcers who require chronic, daily NSAID therapy, patients older than 60 years of age, patients with a history of peptic ulcer disease or GI bleeding, and patients taking concomitant steroids, anticoagulants, or antiplatelets (Chan et al., 2002). The dose of misoprostol is 100 to 200 μg by mouth four times a day, and it should be noted that diarrhea is a common adverse effect of misoprostol that may affect compliance and limit its use in patients. If a patient is considered at very high risk for adverse GI effects because of multiple risk factors or a recent history of ulcer complications, the use of a COX-2 inhibitor plus a PPI is a valuable treatment option. This recommendation is based on the data from a case–control analysis that showed that the use of a COX-2 inhibitor in combination with a PPI was associated with a greater extent of risk reduction of upper GI complications than either a nsNSAID plus a PPI or a COX-2 inhibitor alone. In summary, the strategies for optimizing NSAID therapy in patients with GI risk factors include the use of a nsNSAID with misoprostol, the use of nsNSAID plus a PPI, a COX-2 inhibitor alone, or in the case of very high risk patients, a COX-2 inhibitor with a PPI (Targownik, Metge, Leung, & Chateau, 2008).

In addition to ulcer complications, other GI adverse effects of NSAIDs include dyspepsia, abdominal pain, and heart burn, which affect up to 60% of NSAID users and are associated with significant decrease in quality of life. Dyspepsia symptoms may be alleviated with the addition of a PPI, and taking the NSAID with food may decrease upset stomach in patients.

CV adverse effects

NSAIDs can increase the risk of serious CV thrombotic events, myocardial infarction, and stroke, which can occur as early as the first week of NSAID use and can be fatal (Pepine & Gurbel, 2017; Ruoff, 2015). The risk may be increased with duration of use and in patients with CV disease or risk factors for CV disease. NSAID use is contraindicated for the treatment of perioperative pain in the setting of coronary artery bypass graft surgery (Ruoff, 2015). These CV risk warnings are included in the package insert for all OTC and prescription NSAIDs except aspirin. The selective COX-2 inhibitors can increase the risk of CV events from thromboxane A_2–mediated vasoconstriction and platelet aggregation, which will remain unbalanced and unopposed when prostacyclin activity is suppressed via COX-2 inhibition (Scheiman & Hindley, 2010). The American Heart Association recommends that all NSAIDs should be used at their lowest effective dose and that all NSAIDs, particularly COX-2 selective agents, should be avoided where possible in patients with CV risk factors such as hypertension, hypercholesterolemia, angina, edema, recent bypass surgery, and history of myocardial infarction or other CV events (Antman et al., 2007). NSAIDs should only be used when pain relief is not achieved with other analgesic therapy and benefit outweighs the increased CV risk. It should not be considered that a relative lack of COX-2 selectivity of an NSAID eliminates the risk of CV events as evidenced by the Prospective Randomized Evaluation of Celecoxib Integrated Safety versus Ibuprofen or Naproxen (PRECISION) trial that demonstrated comparable CV safety for celecoxib with naproxen and ibuprofen (Nissen et al., 2016).

Other NSAID adverse effects

Renal complications may occur because of reduced synthesis of PGI2, resulting in signs and symptoms such as peripheral edema, sodium retention, hyperkalemia, and acute renal failure. NSAIDs may increase bleeding risk because of irreversible inhibition of platelet aggregation with aspirin and reversible inhibition of platelet

Table 7–3. Recommendations for the Use of NSAIDs Based on Gastrointestinal and Cardiovascular Risk Factors

No CV Risk Without Aspirin and No or Low GI Risk with NSAID Use	No CV Risk Without Aspirin and GI Risk with NSAID Use
nsNSAID	• COX-2 inhibitor **OR** • nsNSAID + PPI or misoprostol **OR** • COX-2 inhibitor + PPI for those with history of GI bleed
CV Risk on Aspirin and No or Low GI Risk with NSAID Use	**CV Risk on Aspirin and GI Risk with NSAID Use**
• Non-COX-2 selective NSAIDs with lowest GI side effect • Acetaminophen, tramadol, narcotic analgesics (short term) if NSAIDs' CV and GI risks outweigh the benefit • Addition of PPI or misoprostol for GI protection and aspirin 81 mg to prevent thrombotic events	• Acetaminophen, tramadol, narcotic analgesics (short term) if NSAIDs' CV and GI risks outweigh the benefit • Non-COX-2-selective NSAIDs with lowest GI side effect if CV risk outweighs GI • Lowest dose of COX-2 inhibitor if history of GI bleeding • + PPI irrespective of NSAID chosen

COX, cyclooxygenase; CV, cardiovascular; GI, gastrointestinal; NSAID, nonsteroidal anti-inflammatory; nsNSAID, nonselective NSAID; PPI, proton pump inhibitor.
Adapted from Antman, E. M., Bennett, J. S., Daughterty, A., Furberg, C., Roberts, H., & Taubert, K. A. (2007). Use of nonsteroidal anti-inflammatory drugs. An update for clinicians. A statement from the American Heart Association. *Circulation, 115*, 1634–1642; Scheiman, J. M., & Hindley, C., E. (2010). Strategies to optimize treatment with NSAIDs in patients at risk for gastrointestinal and cardiovascular adverse events. *Clinical Therapeutics, 32*, 667–676.

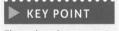

▶ KEY POINT

The major adverse events associated with NSAID use are GI, CV, and renal.

aggregation with the other NSAIDs. Other adverse effects include headache, vertigo, dizziness, confusion, depression, tocolysis in the uterus, and hypersensitivity reactions (Candido, Perozo, & Knezevic, 2017). Pregnant women should avoid NSAIDs in the third trimester of pregnancy because of fetal harm. Table 7-3 provides a summary of the recommendations for NSAID use in patients with GI and CV risk factors.

Acetaminophen

Acetaminophen possesses analgesic and antipyretic properties with very weak anti-inflammatory effect. It inhibits COX-1 and COX-2 centrally and peripherally, resulting in the inhibition of PG synthesis from arachidonic acid. Other proposed analgesic mechanisms of action for acetaminophen may include the endogenous cannabinoid system and inhibition of N-methyl-D-aspartate (NMDA) receptors (Aminoshariae & Khan, 2015). It is useful for mild to moderate pain and is considered a first-line analgesic because of overall safety profile and tolerability. Acetaminophen has a favorable pharmacokinetic profile with 98% bioavailability and onset of analgesia in 30 minutes. Unlike NSAIDs, it is safe for use in patients with renal dysfunction and high blood pressure. It is also considered to be safe for pregnant women. Acetaminophen is also available as intravenous (IV) formulation that can be administered to prevent postoperative pain in addition to decreasing postoperative opioid consumption (Candido et al., 2017).

Adverse Effects of Acetaminophen

Liver toxicity

Hepatotoxicity is the most serious adverse effect associated with acetaminophen, and it occurs in situations of acute overdoses of 7 to 10 g in adults or 150 mg/kg for children and nearly 50% of acetaminophen-related acute liver failure is the result of an unintentional overdose (Aminoshariae & Khan, 2015). Acetaminophen at therapeutic doses may also cause hepatotoxicity if patients have risk factors such as chronic alcohol ingestion and malnutrition or acute starvation. Many products contain acetaminophen, including OTC pain cough-and-cold products and prescription pain medications. Thus, it is essential to be aware of all the medication products that patients may be taking that contain acetaminophen to avoid unintentional overdoses. The maximum daily dose for acetaminophen is 4 g, and in patients with liver disease, the maximum daily dose decreases to 2 g (Aminoshariae & Khan, 2015).

Other adverse effects of acetaminophen

Exposure to acetaminophen may increase the risk of asthma and wheezing in children. There is cross-sensitivity between aspirin and acetaminophen in aspirin-sensitive asthmatic patients (Aminoshariae & Khan, 2015).

 ▶ KEY POINT

Adverse effects associated with acetaminophen are mainly hepatotoxicity and cross-sensitivity.

Opioid Analgesics

Opioid analgesics act by binding to opioid receptors of three subtypes: mu, kappa, and delta. Mu opioid receptors are located along the nociceptive pathway, and the analgesic effect of opioids occurs through agonism at mu opioid receptors with a resultant decrease in afferent nociceptive neuronal depolarization. Opioids may be classified by their chemical classes or their actions as agonist, agonist/antagonist (partial agonist), or antagonist (Table 7-4) (Jamison & Mao, 2015; Trescot, Datta,

Table 7-4. Chemical Classes of Opioids

Phenanthrenes	**Agonist:** morphine, codeine, oxycodone, hydromorphone, oxymorphone, hydrocodone, levorphanol **Partial agonist:** buprenorphine, butorphanol, nalbuphine
Phenylpiperidines	**Agonist:** fentanyl (highest affinity for mu receptor), alfentanil, sufentanil, meperidine
Diphenylheptane	**Agonist:** methadone (also antagonist at N-methyl-D-aspartate receptor)
Benzomorphans	**Partial agonist:** pentazocine (a high incidence of dysphoria)
Other Opioids	
Atypical Opioid	Tramadol, tapentadol

Adapted from Trescot, A. M., Datta, S., Lee, M., & Hansen, H. (2008). Opioid pharmacology. *Pain Physician, 11,* S133–S153.

Lee, & Hansen, 2008). Opioids are commonly used to treat moderate-to-severe acute pain, cancer-related chronic pain, and pain at the end of life. Their role in the treatment of chronic noncancer pain is controversial and should be managed by a pain specialist that can pay attention to pain, function, adverse effects in addition to signs of abuse and addiction. Guidelines for using opioids for chronic noncancer pain have been released by the Centers for Disease Control and Prevention in 2016 (Dowell, Haegerich, & Chou, 2016) and should be followed when prescribing, administering, and dispensing opioids.

Opioids have differences in opioid potency but all mu opioid agonists are considered to be equally effective analgesics when used at equivalent doses. The choice of opioid analgesic is based on patient and drug-specific factors such as organ function, dosage form, and cost. There is no ceiling dose for opioids, and the maximum dose is limited only by side effects.

Morphine, oxycodone, hydromorphone, and fentanyl are the most commonly used opioids. Methadone is also used for the treatment of pain but because of its complex pharmacokinetic properties and unique safety considerations, it is only used by experienced pain specialists. There are many formulations available for opioids including oral, IV, transdermal, subcutaneous, sublingual, intranasal, buccal, and suppositories. This section will discuss the characteristics that are unique for each of the opioids and the factors that should be taken into consideration when these agents are being prescribed and administered to patients for pain management.

Codeine is a prodrug of morphine and requires metabolism by cytochrome P450 2D6 (CYP2D6) enzyme in the liver to morphine, norcodeine (via CYP3A4), and codeine-6-glucuronide (Trescot et al., 2008). Only about 10% of codeine is metabolized to morphine, and codeine has half the analgesic potency of morphine. Genetic polymorphisms of the metabolic enzyme CYP2D6 produce three population phenotypes: extensive metabolizer (EM), ultra-rapid metabolizer (UM), and poor metabolizer (PM). When a patient is initiated on an adequate dose of codeine and does not seem to experience analgesia, the patient may be a PM of codeine. Patients with the UM phenotype produce approximately 50% more morphine compared to EM; therefore, if a patient is experiencing severe side effects such as sedation or respiratory depression on an average dose of codeine, consider that the patient may be an UM of the drug. In fact, codeine has a black box warning in the package insert warning against prescribing to children because of the unknown potential of the child being an UM and with increased risk of toxic adverse effects. Breastfeeding mothers who are CYP2D6 UM and are taking codeine for analgesia may put infants at increased risk for potentially life-threatening central nervous system (CNS) depression. Thus, it is important to ensure that nursing mothers who are prescribed codeine receive the lowest effective dose or, if at all possible, avoid codeine. Drug interactions with codeine occur when codeine is taken concomitantly with drugs that are inhibitors or inducers of the CYP2D6 or CYP3A4 enzymes. Codeine is available as a single agent and in combination with acetaminophen or aspirin for pain indications. Doses of codeine greater than 65 mg are not well tolerated. Paradoxically, codeine is more emetogenic at lower doses compared to higher doses possibly because of competing effect at the chemoreceptor trigger zone (Trescot et al., 2008).

Hydrocodone is similar in structure to codeine and it displays weak binding capacity at the mu opioid receptor (Trescot et al., 2008). Hydrocodone is metabolized by CYP2D6 to hydromorphone, which has stronger binding at the mu opioid receptor than hydrocodone. It is available as a combination product with either ibuprofen or acetaminophen and as extended release single-agent hydrocodone. In the combination formulation, the dose of the hydrocodone is limited by the nonopioid analgesic, which has a ceiling maximum dose.

Morphine is the standard of comparison for all opioid drugs. Based on clinicians' familiarity with its use and availability in multiple formulations (including oral, rectal, IV, subcutaneous, intrathecal, intranasal, sustained release, and immediate release), morphine is one of the most commonly prescribed opioid analgesics for the management of pain. Morphine is predominantly metabolized in the liver by glucuronidation to produce morphine-3-glucuronide (M3G) and morphine-6-glucuronide (M6G). M6G is an active metabolite that possesses greater analgesic effect compared to its parent compound, morphine, and M6G is also associated with opioid adverse effects. In contrast, the M3G metabolite is primarily associated with side effects with no analgesic effect. The morphine metabolites are excreted renally; thus, accumulation of the metabolites may occur in patients with renal dysfunction and cause prolonged side effects. Consider avoiding morphine and using opioids that are not renally eliminated in patients with renal insufficiency. The extended release morphine may be administered every 24 hours (e.g., Avinza), every 12 to 24 hours (e.g., Kadian), or every 8 to 12 hours (e.g., Oramorph, MS contin, generic morphine extended release). The extended release morphine is to be taken whole and must not be broken, chewed, or crushed to prevent potential toxicity (Prommer, 2015b; Trescot et al., 2008).

Oxycodone possesses analgesic potency that is 1.5 times as potent as morphine (Prommer, 2015b). It is available as a single agent or in combination with acetaminophen, ibuprofen, or aspirin. Oxycodone only exists as capsules, tablets, or solution for oral administration. There is a ceiling maximum dose with the combination product because of the nonopioid component. The extended release formulation of oxycodone has indications for every 12 hours dosing; however, in clinical practice, some patients may require every 8 hours dosing for optimal pain control. Ten percent of oxycodone is metabolized by CYP2D6 to the active metabolite oxymorphone; however, oxycodone is not a prodrug and it possesses analgesic activity (Trescot et al., 2008).

Hydromorphone is about 7 to 11 times more potent than morphine (Trescot et al., 2008). Hydromorphone is metabolized to hydromorphone-3-glucuronide that has no analgesic effect but is associated with neuroexcitatory side effects such as allodynia, myoclonus, confusion, and seizures. There are no reported drug–drug interactions with this drug. Hydromorphone has oral, parenteral, intraspinal, and suppository formulations. It is available as immediate release and single, daily dose, extended release oral formulation. The duration of analgesic effect for immediate release hydromorphone is shorter than morphine or oxycodone, lasting around 2 to 3 hours (Prommer, 2015b; Trescot et al., 2008).

Oxymorphone is a metabolite of oxycodone and it is approximately 10 times more potent than morphine. It is available as immediate or extended release oral formulations and parenteral formulations. The immediate release oral formulation has a longer half-life (7.2-9.4 hours) than most immediate release opioids; therefore, every 6 hours dosing is recommended for short-acting oxymorphone compared to every 4 hours for other short-acting opioids (Prommer, 2015b). Oxymorphone is excreted by the kidneys and dose adjustment or switching to opioids that are not renally eliminated should be considered for patients with renal dysfunction. In patients with hepatic insufficiency, the dosing interval should be increased (Prommer, 2015b).

Fentanyl is a synthetic opioid analgesic that is 100 times more potent than morphine. Fentanyl is very lipophilic, which allows absorption of the drug through the skin and mucous membranes en route to the systemic circulation (Prommer, 2015b). Fentanyl is available as transdermal, parenteral, and transmucosal products. The transmucosal formulations of fentanyl are indicated for breakthrough pain, in opioid-tolerant patients. When applying the transdermal fentanyl patch, it is important to note that it has a lag time of 12 hours to onset of analgesic effect; it takes 12 to 24 hours before serum concentrations stabilize, and it takes 3 to 6 days before steady-state concentration is reached (Trescot et al., 2008). The recommended dosing for the patch is every 72 hours; however, some patients may require every 48 hours dosing. Based on its pharmacokinetic profile, the patch is not initiated for management of acute pain but is usually considered once a patient has reached a stable pain level with shorter-acting analgesics and is switched to the fentanyl patch. Because of the lag time for onset of analgesic effect, it is recommended that there is overlapping of the shorter-acting opioid dose with the patch for about 12 hours prior to discontinuation of the shorter-acting agent.

Methadone is a synthetic mu- and delta opioid receptor agonist; it also causes monoamine reuptake inhibition and possesses antagonist activity at the NMDA receptor (Trescot et al., 2008). Methadone is a racemic mixture of two enantiomers, the R form is more potent with a 10-fold higher affinity for the opioid receptor. The S form inhibits reuptake of serotonin and norepinephrine and is antagonistic at the NMDA receptor. It is thought that the NMDA antagonistic effect of methadone makes it a useful agent for the treatment of neuropathic pain. Methadone is a highly lipid-soluble drug that is redistributed to fat tissue, resulting in erratic pharmacokinetics with a long plasma half-life of approximately 24 hours (range, 12-150 hours). Because of the unpredictable long elimination half-life and the potential for drug accumulation in tissues causing delayed toxicities, the use of methadone for the treatment of pain requires vigilant monitoring during initiation and dose titration of the drug. Steady state is not achieved for approximately 2 weeks after therapy initiation or dose change; therefore, the patient should be on a dose for at least 5 to 7 days before deciding to increase the dose again for ineffective pain relief. Although the drug has a long half-life, the analgesic effect is only 4 to 6 hours; thus, the dosing interval for methadone for pain management is every 6 to 8 hours and may be increased to every 8 to 12 hours with chronic use. It is available in formulations for oral and parenteral administration. The tablet may be crushed and dissolved for nasogastric tube administration or the oral solution may be used. It is metabolized by the liver and excreted primarily in the feces. Despite its limitations, advantages of methadone include its cost-effectiveness, safety in renal insufficiency, and convenience of every 6 to 8 hours dosing frequency. Methadone is metabolized by CYP3A4, CYP2D6, and CYP2B6 enzymes. There is a potential association between CYP3A inhibitor drug interaction and methadone-induced torsades de pointes. Drug–drug interactions with methadone should be carefully evaluated when drugs that are CYP3A4 inhibitors or inducers are in a patient's medication profile. Methadone has the potential to initiate torsades de pointes, causing a lengthening of the QT interval and resulting in possible fatal arrhythmias. Factors that increase the risk for torsades de pointes include congenital QT prolongation, methadone doses over 60 mg per day, hypokalemia, and hypomagnesemia. Patients should be closely monitored for torsades de pointes and a baseline electrocardiogram is recommended for high-risk patients (Prommer, 2015b; Trescot et al., 2008).

Tramadol and **tapentadol** bind weakly to mu opioid receptors, inhibit the reuptake of serotonin and norepinephrine, and promote neuronal serotonin release; thus, they share pharmacologic properties of opioids and tricyclic antidepressants (TCAs). Caution is advised when either agent is administered with selective serotonin reuptake inhibitors, monoamine oxidase inhibitors, or TCAs because of the risk of serotonin syndrome. It is believed that tramadol and tapentadol have low abuse potential and low risk of respiratory depression. Toxic doses of tramadol and tapentadol can result in CNS excitation and seizures. Tramadol is available as immediate release combination product with acetaminophen or as a single agent, and as controlled release formulation (Trescot et al., 2008). Tramadol is metabolized by CYP2D6 to its active metabolite that contributes to analgesia; patients who are PMs of CYP2D6 may experience poor analgesia. Concurrent administration of CYP2D6 inhibitors and tramadol should be avoided if possible to prevent inadequate analgesia. Tapentadol, on the other hand, does not require metabolism for its analgesic effect and it has no active metabolites. Tapentadol is available as immediate and extended release formulations.

Buprenorphine is a partial agonist with very high affinity for the mu opioid receptor and does not get displaced easily by an antagonist such as naloxone. When reversal of buprenorphine is necessary, it may require high doses of an antagonist for a prolonged period of time. Furthermore, buprenorphine can displace pure μ-agonist drugs like morphine off the opioid receptor and induce withdrawal. This is a concern when patients are being switched from another opioid to buprenorphine (Chen, Chen, & Mao, 2014). There is a ceiling analgesic effect with buprenorphine because it is a partial agonist; however, there is a ceiling effect for respiratory depression at high doses of buprenorphine that is independent of the analgesic effect; therefore, it may be a safe alternative for patients who are predisposed to respiratory problems. Buprenorphine is metabolized in the liver by CYP3A4 to norbuprenorphine, a weak active metabolite. There is potential for drug–drug interactions with inducers and inhibitors of CYP3A4. The metabolite passes into the bile and is excreted through feces, which makes it safe for administration in patients with renal insufficiency. Buprenorphine is available in parenteral, oral, sublingual, and transdermal formulations. The sublingual formulation is for the treatment of opioid dependence, not for the treatment of pain. Buprenorphine is also formulated in conjunction with naloxone as a film to be administered sublingually for the treatment of opioid dependence. The naloxone is not absorbed sublingually or orally but, instead, the intent is to reverse the effect of parenteral opioid administration that may be attempted (Trescot et al., 2008). Buprenorphine is available as a patch for transdermal administration that is indicated for moderate-to-severe chronic pain when continuous, around-the-clock opioid analgesic is needed for an extended period of time. Buprenorphine patch is applied and removed every 7 days. Do not exceed a dose of 20 µg/h because of the risk for QTc prolongation (Prommer, 2015a).

▊ Adverse Effects of Opioids

Opioids produce a broad spectrum of adverse effects including euphoria, dysphoria, constipation, nausea, vomiting, pruritus because of histamine release, sedation, respiratory depression, suppression of endocrine systems, bradycardia, seizures, and miosis. Constipation is the most persistent adverse effect that worsens with duration of use and increasing dose. Patients should be counseled to take laxatives such as polyethylene glycol and senokot on a scheduled basis with the commencement of opioid analgesics to prevent constipation. The patient develops tolerance to the other adverse effects and it diminishes over days to weeks of exposure.

▊ Adjuvant Analgesics

Adjuvant analgesics are agents that are useful in the management of pain though they are not classified as analgesics. They include antiepileptic medications, antidepressants, and topical anesthetics. These agents can be added to opioid or nonopioid analgesics as part of a multimodal pain management approach usually to treat neuropathic pain. A therapeutic effect of adjuvant analgesics is that it has a dose-sparing effect on opioids, which reduces opioid side effects and adds a different mechanism of action in opioid-resistant pain. Adjuvant analgesics have a narrow therapeutic window and the higher the dose, the greater the likelihood of side effects. There is a ceiling effect in which there is no further pain relief above a specific dose.

Gabapentin and pregabalin bind to the $\alpha_2\delta$ subunit of voltage-gated Ca^{2+} channels causing modulation of cellular calcium influx into nociceptive neurons. This results in reduction in neurotransmitter release and decrease in neuronal hyperexcitability (Hendrich et al., 2008). The dose for gabapentin should start low at 100 mg three times daily and may be increased by 300 mg daily until pain relief is achieved or the maximum dose of 3,600 mg a day is reached. Bioavailability of gabapentin is reduced from 60% to 33% as doses are increased from 900 to 3,600 mg daily. For patients not responding to gabapentin (at doses >900 mg a day), a switch to pregabalin or duloxetine or the addition of duloxetine to gabapentin may improve pain control (Davis, 2018). The initial dose for pregabalin is 50 or 75 mg twice daily and can be escalated by 50 to 75 mg every 1 to 2 days up to a maximum of 600 mg a day in two divided doses. Pregabalin has 90% bioavailability and does not change with increasing dose. The dose of pregabalin and gabapentin needs to be adjusted in patients with renal impairment. The side effects for gabapentin and pregabalin are similar and include sedation, dizziness, and peripheral edema.

TCA and serotonin and norepinephrine reuptake inhibitors (SNRIs) have demonstrated efficacy in patients with neuropathic pain. They block NMDA receptors and sodium channels, block uptake of spinal noradrenaline and adenosine, resulting in modulation of descending inhibitory pathways. The dose (initial dose of 10–25 mg at night) of the TCA for neuropathic pain is lower than that used to treat depression (Binder & Baron, 2016). They are helpful for neuropathic pain in patients with insomnia. Amitriptyline, imipramine, desipramine, and nortriptyline have been used with preference for desipramine and nortriptyline because of fewer anticholinergic effects. The SNRIs that are used for neuropathic pain include venlafaxine and duloxetine. The starting dose for venlafaxine is 37.5 mg orally daily and doubled weekly. The doses of venlafaxine for noradrenaline reuptake inhibition is 150 to 225 mg. Initial doses for duloxetine are 20 to 30 mg daily, increasing to 60 mg daily a week later. Doses of 60 mg per day improve neuropathic pain and there are no benefits with doses of 120 mg (Binder & Baron, 2016). Side effects for venlafaxine include hypertension and QTC prolongation. For duloxetine, side effects include nausea, headache, dizziness, dry mouth, constipation, and hyperhidrosis. Duloxetine does not have the cardiac side effects that venlafaxine and TCAs have (Binder & Baron, 2016). Tricyclics should not be combined with SNRI because of increased risk of serotonin syndrome.

Topical lidocaine relieves pain through nonspecific block of sodium channels on ectopic peripheral afferent fibers. The 5% lidocaine patch is recommended for localized peripheral neuropathic pain. Initial dose is one to three patches to the painful area for 12 hours, with application-free interval for 12 hours, with a maximum of three patches in 24 hours.

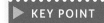
▶ **KEY POINT**

Adjuvant analgesics include antiepileptic medications, antidepressants, and topical anesthetics.

▌ Summary

Pain is a main reason patients seek medical advice and pain management is enhanced when a multimodal pharmacologic approach is utilized to maximize efficacy and minimize adverse effects. Understanding the pathophysiology of pain and aligning this with the appropriate analgesic agent for the treatment of the pain diagnosis are important steps in addressing pain control. Furthermore, knowing the pharmacokinetic and adverse effect profile of the pharmacologic agents will further facilitate the decision process in choosing the optimal drug regimen for a patient.

REFERENCES

Aminoshariae, A., & Khan, A. (2015). Acetaminophen: Old drug, new issues. *Journal of Endodontics, 41*, 588–593.

Antman, E. M., Bennett, J. S., Daughterty, A., Furberg, C., Roberts, H., & Taubert, K. A. (2007). Use of nonsteroidal anti-inflammatory drugs. An update for clinicians. A statement from the American Heart Association. *Circulation, 115*, 1634–1642.

Bacchi, S., Palumbo, P., Sponta, A., & Coppolino, M. F. (2012). Clinical pharmacology of non-steroidal anti-inflammatory drugs: A review. *Anti-Inflammatory & Anti-Allergy Agents in Medicinal Chemistry, 11*, 52–64.

Bardou M., & Barkun A. N. (2010). Preventing the gastrointestinal adverse effects of nonsteroidal anti-inflammatory drugs: From risk factor identification to risk factor intervention. *Joint Bone Spine, 77*, 6–12.

Binder, A., & Baron, R. (2016). The pharmacological therapy of chronic neuropathic pain. *Deutsches Ärzteblatt International, 113*(37), 616–625.

Candido, K. D., Perozo, O. J., & Knezevic, N. N. (2017). Pharmacology of acetaminophen, non-steroidal anti-inflammatory drugs, and steroidal medications: Implications for anesthesia or unique associated risks. *Anesthesiology Clinic, 35*, e145–e162.

Chan, F. K., Hung, L. C., Suen, B. Y., Wu, J. C., Lee, K. C., Leung, V. K., . . . Sung J. J. (2002). Celecoxib versus diclofenac and omeprazole in reducing the risk of recurrent ulcer bleeding in patients with arthritis. *New England Journal of Medicine, 347*, 2104–2110.

Chen K. Y., Chen L., & Mao J. (2014). Buprenorphine-naloxone therapy in pain management. *Anesthesiology, 120*, 1262–1274.

Dhillon, S. (2011). Naproxen/esomeprazole fixed-dose combination: For the treatment of arthritic symptoms and to reduce the risk of gastric ulcers. *Drugs & Aging, 28*, 237–248.

Dowell, D., Haegerich, T. M., & Chou, R. (2016). CDC guideline for prescribing opioids for chronic pain – United States, 2016. *The Journal of the American Medical Association, 315*(15), 1624–1645.

Goldstein, J. L., Hochberg, M. C., Fort, J. C., Zhang, Y., Hwang, C., & Sostek, M. (2010). Clinical trial: The incidence of NSAID-associated endoscopic gastric ulcers in patients treated with PN 400 (naproxen plus esomeprazole magnesium) vs. enteric coated naproxen alone. *Alimentary Pharmacology & Therapeutics, 32*, 401–413.

Hendrich, J., Van Minh, A. T., Heblich, F., Nieto-Rostro, M., Watschinger, K., Striessnig, J... Dolphin, A. C. (2008). Pharmacological disruption of calcium channel trafficking by the alpha2delta ligand gabapentin. Proceedings of the National Acadies of Science, 105(9), 3628–3633.

Huntjens, D. R. H., Danhof, M., & Della Pasqua, O. E. (2005). Pharmacokinetic-pharmacodynamic correlations and biomarkers in the development of COX-2 inhibitors. *Rheumatology, 44*, 846–859.

Jamison R. N., & Mao, J. (2015). Opioid analgesics. *Mayo Clinic Proceedings, 90*, 957–968.

Laine, L., Kivitz, A. J., Bello, A. E., Grahn, A. Y., Schiff, M. H., & Taha, A. S. (2012). Double-blind randomized trials of single-tablet ibuprofen/high-dose famotidine vs. ibuprofen alone for reduction of gastric and duodenal ulcers. *American Journal of Gastroenterology, 107*, 379–386.

Lanza, F. L., Chan, F. K., Quigley, E. M., & The Practice Parameters Committee of the American College of Gastroenterology. (2009). Guidelines for prevention of NSAID-related ulcer complications. *American Journal of Gastroenterology, 104*, 728–738.

McPherson, M. L., & Cimino, N. M. (2013). Topical NSAID formulations. *Pain Medicine, 14*, S35–S39.

Meara, A. S., & Simon, L. S. (2013). Advice from professional societies: Appropriate use of NSAIDs. *Pain Medicine, 14*, S3–S10.

Nissen, S. E., Yeomans, N. D., Solomon, D. H., Luscher, T. F., Libby, P., Husni, M. E, ...Lincoff, A. M. (2016). Cardiovascular safety of celecoxib, naproxen, or ibuprofen for arthritis. *New England Journal of Medicine, 375*, 2519–2529.

Pepine, C. J., & Gurbel, P. A. (2017). Cardiovascular safety of NSAIDs: Additional insights after PRECISION and point of view. *Clinical Cardiology, 40*, 1352–1356.

Prommer, E. (2015a). Buprenorphine for cancer pain: Is it ready for prime time? *American Journal of Hospice & Palliative Medicine, 32*, 881–889.

Prommer, E. E. (2015b). Pharmacological management of cancer related pain. *Cancer Control, 22*, 412–422.

Ruoff, G. (2015). Nonsteroidal anti-inflammatory drugs and cardiovascular risk: Where are we today? *The Journal of Family Practice, 64*, S67–S70.

Scheiman, J. M., & Hindley, C., E. (2010). Strategies to optimize treatment with NSAIDs in patients at risk for gastrointestinal and cardiovascular adverse events. *Clinical Therapeutics, 32*, 667–676.

Simon, L. S., & Strand, V. (1997). Clinical response to nonsteroidal anti-inflammatory drugs. *Arthritis & Rheumatism, 40,* 1940–1943.

Targownik, L. E., Metge, C. J., Leung, S., & Chateau, D. G. (2008). The relative efficacies of gastroprotective strategies in chronic users of nonsteroidal anti-inflammatory drugs. *Gastroenterology, 134,* 937–944.

Theken, K. N. (2018). Variability in analgesic response to non-steroidal anti-inflammatory drugs. *Prostaglandins and Other Lipid Mediators, 139,* 63–70.

Trescot, A. M., Datta, S., Lee, M., & Hansen, H. (2008). Opioid pharmacology. *Pain Physician, 11,* S133–S153.

Warner, T. D., Giuliano, F., Vojnovic, I., Bukasa, A., Mitchell, J. A., & Vane, J. R. (1999). Nonsteroidal rug selectivities for cyclo-oxygenase-1 rather than cyclo-oxygenase-2 are associated with human gastrointestinal toxicity: A full *in vitro* analysis. *Proceedings of the National Academy of Sciences, 96,* 7563–7568.

Wickham, R. (2017). Cancer pain management: Comprehensive assessment and nonopioid analgesics, part I. *Journal of the Advanced Practitioner in Oncology, 8,* 475–490.

CHAPTER 8

NON-PHARMACOLOGIC MANAGEMENT OF PAIN

Deborah Dillon McDonald

Non-pharmacologic management of pain is an essential aspect of pain management. Although non-pharmacologic strategies may be used as primary treatment without the use of medication or supplements, they are often used along with, or complementary to, pharmacologic treatment to facilitate effective pain management.

Complementary pain treatments encompass adjuvant pain treatments not routinely prescribed in Western healthcare (National Center for Complementary and Integrative Health [NCCIH], 2018a). The terms "integrative" and "alternative" are also used to describe complementary treatments, with the former including both traditional Western and complementary treatments and the latter including only complementary treatments (NCCIH, 2018a). Although complementary treatments include dietary supplements such as glucosamine, only nondietary complementary pain treatments are reviewed in this chapter. Spinal manipulation is considered by some to be a complementary treatment (NCCIH, 2018b), but is not included in the review because it is an established part of Western healthcare (NCCIH, 2018c). For a review of complementary pain treatments that include nutritional supplements and spinal manipulation, see Nahin, Boineau, Khalsa, Stussman, and Weber (2016). Finally, exercise such as walking is commonly prescribed to reduce pain in Western healthcare and as a result is not included in the review. This chapter provides an overview of research evidence of complementary pain treatments used by adults for acupuncture, massage, tai chi, yoga, mindfulness, and music. The reviewed research evidence consisted almost exclusively of meta-analyses of randomized controlled trials (RCTs).

Complementary pain treatments offer the potential for decreased pain without adverse drug responses, although adverse treatment responses remain possible. An estimated 33.2% of adults in the United States use complementary treatments (Clarke, Black, Stussman, Barnes, &

> ▶ **KEY POINT**
>
> Complementary pain treatments offer the potential for decreased pain without adverse drug responses. Research supports each of the six reviewed complementary pain treatments (acupuncture, massage, tai chi, yoga, mindfulness, and music) as efficacious for at least one pain condition in adults and some pain conditions respond to multiple complementary pain treatments.

Nahin, 2015), many for pain self-management. The estimated annual out-of-pocket cost for complementary pain treatment is $14.9 billion, with $8.7 billion used for back pain alone (Nahin, Stussman, & Herman, 2015). Increased use of complementary pain treatments requires that practitioners understand which complementary pain treatments are empirically supported for specific pain conditions.

Acupuncture

Acupuncture is a traditional Chinese medicine technique that involves procedures to stimulate points on the body. Acupuncture frequently involves penetrating the skin with metallic acupuncture needles (NCCIH, 2018d). Acupuncture has been examined across a wide range of pain conditions from treatment of acute pain in the emergency room to chronic low back pain and cancer-related pain.

Meta-analysis of 14 RCTs supported acupuncture for several acute pain conditions treated in the emergency department. Acupuncture reduced fracture pain the most with a large standard mean difference (SMD) of 2.06 (confidence interval [CI] = 1.43-2.69), had a medium effect on acute back pain with an SMD of 0.75 (CI = 0.03 to −1.48), a medium effect for migraine pain with an SMD of 0.60 (CI = 0.18-1.03), and a small effect for renal colic pain with an SMD of −0.21 (CI = −0.86 to 0.43). Acupuncture reduced acute pain to a level similar to analgesics and when coadministered with analgesics produced an additive effect. Ear acupuncture had a greater effect on pain reduction than acupuncture at other sites; however, no direct comparisons were made. Research that used the same acupoints without needle penetration as the comparison group had a medium, but smaller effect than research without an acupoint comparison group, perhaps because of more rigorous control of response bias. Adverse effects from acupuncture were relatively low at 5.04%. Heterogeneity (high variability) among the studies included in the meta-analysis remains a concern, however (Jan et al., 2017).

Acupuncture for the treatment of acute surgical pain after back surgery has been supported in a subanalysis of two RCTs within a five RCT meta-analysis. Both studies were from the same investigators. Results supported a moderate effect size of acupuncture on reduced pain intensity with an SMD of −0.67 (CI = −1.04 to −0.31) with no heterogeneity concerns (Cho et al., 2015), providing clearer evidence that acupuncture reduces acute surgical pain.

The effect of acupuncture in treating osteoarthritis pain in adults was examined in a meta-analysis of 12 RCTs. Only three of the RCTs had low risk of bias. Combination of the three trials with a total of 410 adults supported a mean pain intensity reduction of −0.59 (CI = −1.18 to −0.0). Comparison of length of intervention across six RCTs dichotomized as less than 4 weeks and 4 weeks and greater supported that longer duration interventions resulted in a greater reduction in pain intensity, SMD −0.38 (CI = −0.69 to −0.06). Functional mobility was also significantly increased as a result of the acupuncture, along with health-related quality of life (Manyanga et al., 2014).

Treatment of nonspecific chronic low back pain with acupuncture is cautiously supported by meta-analysis results. Subanalysis of 5 studies from a 25-study meta-analysis for the effect of acupuncture on nonspecific chronic low back pain supported that acupuncture compared to no treatment produced a moderate effect of SMD of −0.72 (CI = −0.94 to −0.49) immediately posttreatment. Furthermore, across four studies, acupuncture compared to sham treatment resulted in a mean 100 mm visual analog scale score reduction of −16.76 (CI = −33.33 to −0.19) (Lam, Galvin, & Curry, 2013). High heterogeneity among the studies and small pooled sample sizes demand cautious interpretation, however.

Acupuncture provides moderate pain reduction for malignancy-related pain, with an effect size of −0.71 (CI = −0.94 to −0.048) as reported in a meta-analysis of 29 RCTs of acupuncture and cancer-related pain. Acupuncture more modestly reduced acute surgical pain after cancer surgery with an effect of −0.40 (CI = −0.69 to −0.10). Results must be interpreted within the context of risk for bias across all studies, unclear description of acupuncture procedures, and wide variability in outcomes (Chiu, Hsieh, & Tsai, 2016). Acupuncture as treatment for pain associated with aromatase inhibitor–induced arthralgia was supported in studies using the Western Ontario and McMaster Universities Arthritis Index (WOMAC) but not the Brief Pain Inventory. Reduction in pain intensity occurred after 6 to 8 weeks of acupuncture treatment (Chen et al., 2017).

Acupuncture for pain reduction from dysmenorrhea was examined in a meta-analysis that included 49 RCTs. As with previous meta-analyses of acupuncture for pain treatment, heterogeneity was a problem. Subanalysis of five studies using the visual analog scale supported that manual acupuncture resulted in a significant reduction in pain intensity, SMD = −1.22 (CI = −1.53 to −0.91), after 180 minutes in a sample of 210 women (Woo et al., 2018).

Laser acupuncture involves laser rather than manual stimulation with needles. For musculoskeletal pain, meta-analysis of 33 RCTs supported a small reduction in pain intensity of SMD = −0.43 (CI = −0.74 to −0.12) at short-term follow-up after laser acupuncture, and a moderate effect of SMD = −0.61 (CI = −1.12 to −0.10) at long-term follow-up when laser acupuncture was compared to placebo conditions. No significant pain reduction was supported in RCTs comparing laser acupuncture to control conditions. High heterogeneity among the included studies and dose and time to effect are all areas that require further examination to guide use of laser acupuncture as an effective pain treatment (Law, McDonough, Bleakley, Baxter, & Tumilty, 2015).

Massage

Massage involves the use of hands to systematically manipulate soft tissue with the aim of producing positive effects that can include pain reduction (Crawford et al., 2016). Massage to reduce pain has been studied in acute and chronic pain conditions, and more specifically in postsurgical pain and in cancer-related pain. Meta-analysis of 32 randomized controlled clinical trials testing massage in people with acute or chronic pain supported weak positive evidence that massage reduces pain when compared to a sham or active comparator conditions (e.g., relaxation). When compared to no treatment, massage has a stronger effect in reducing pain. Heterogeneity was high, indicating considerable variability between the combined RCTs, however (Crawford et al., 2016).

Cancer-related pain represents a wide variety of affected body systems and differs further if metastases are present. Thus, heterogeneity remains a common problem when comparing across RCTs. Meta-analysis of six RCTs with a total $n = 370$ supported weak positive evidence from massage compared to an active comparator. Reduction of pain intensity was not clinically significant, and heterogeneity among the RCTs was high (Boyd et al., 2016a), however. A larger meta-analysis with 12 RCTs and $n = 559$ people with cancer-related pain provided sensitivity analyses to further inform clinical practice. Analysis of all 12 studies as well as analysis of the 9 high-quality RCTs supported massage as significantly reducing cancer-related pain. In three RCTs of metastatic cancer–related pain, heterogeneity was acceptable and a significant effect was supported for massage. Breast cancer–related pain was analyzed across four studies and supported massage as significantly reducing pain. Analysis of three studies supported massage as effective 2 weeks after the massage treatment. Pooled results from seven studies supported body massage as effective, pooled results from four studies supported foot reflexology as effective, and pooled results from two studies supported aroma massage as effective in reducing cancer-related pain. Massage dose differed across the RCTs with time $M = 29.5$ minutes (range $= 10$-50 minutes), sessions $M = 4.5$ (range $= 1$-12 sessions), and duration $M = 23.6$ days (range $= 1$-140 days) (Lee, Kim, Yeo, Kim, & Lim, 2015).

Massage as a treatment for acute postoperative pain was examined in two meta-analyses. Meta-analysis of critical or acutely ill adults following thoracic surgery that compared massage to sham or attention control or standard care provided weak evidence for pain reduction when all groups also received analgesics. All but one of the 12 studies exclusively examined coronary artery bypass grafts or valve replacement patients, and the majority of patients were male. High heterogeneity and risk of bias suggest cautious interpretation of the results (Boiter, Gelinas, Richard-Lalonde, & Thombs, 2017). Pain reduction was again supported in a second meta-analysis with seven RCTs ($n = 1101$) across multiple surgical procedures. Results approached clinical significance, with a visual analog scale score reduction of -19.85 (Boyd et al., 2016b).

Tai Chi

Tai chi involves slow and gentle body movements while breathing deeply and med itating on the movement. Different tai chi styles exist such as Yang, Sun and Wu (NCCIH, 2018e). Results from two meta-analyses support tai chi as effective in reducing osteoarthritis pain (Hall et al., 2017; Kong et al., 2016); however, the meta-analyses overlapped and included seven of the same research studies. A moderate short-term effect on osteoarthritis pain reduction occurred across 8 RCTs (SMD $= -0.54$, CI $= -0.77$ to -0.30 [Kong et al., 2016]) and 11 RCTs (SMD $= -0.66$, CI $= -0.85$ to -0.48 [Hall et al., 2017]). Tai chi significantly reduced pain compared to wait-list control and attention control groups, but was not significantly different when compared to active therapy.

Duration of tai chi impacts the pain outcomes. Tai chi duration of 5 weeks or less does not reduce pain, whereas tai chi duration of 6 to 10 weeks results in a moderate pain reduction (SMD $= -0.50$, CI $= 0.83$ to -0.17), and tai chi greater than 10 weeks results in slightly more pain reduction (SMD = −0.57, CI = −0.86 to −0.27) (Kong et al., 2016). Tai chi is therefore a viable complementary pain treatment for osteoarthritis pain when practiced 6 weeks or more.

Yoga

Yoga originated from Indian philosophy and involves mind- and body-focused activities that include specific postures, breathing techniques, and meditation or relaxation. Several different yoga techniques exist and include Hatha, Iyengar, Vinyasa, Bikram, Anusara, and Ashtanga (NCCIH, 2018f).

Meta-analysis results for chronic low back pain outcomes from five RCTs supported that practicing yoga resulted in moderate pain reduction after a yoga treatment regimen (Cohen's d = 0.62, CI = 0.38-0.87) with low heterogeneity (I^2 = 22.4%). The pain reduction declined to a small, but significant value at follow-up (Cohen's d = 0.40, CI = 0.53-0.85); however, heterogeneity was high at I^2 = 74.8% (Holtzman & Beggs, 2013). Types of yoga used in the studies included Hatha, Viniyoga, and Iyengar. Ward, Stebbings, Cherkin, and Baxter's (2013) meta-analysis included four of the five same RCTs and as expected produced similar results (SMD = −0.61, CI = −0.97 to −0.26) for pain intensity after yoga treatment. Yoga regimens generally included 30 minutes per day 4 days/wk. Yoga for chronic low back pain and other common pain conditions was examined in a meta-analysis by Bussing, Ostermann, Ludtke, and Michalsen (2012) that also included studies from the previous meta-analyses. Yoga reduced pain moderately in conditions other than chronic low back pain and rheumatoid arthritis (SMD = −0.54). The effect of yoga on rheumatoid arthritis pain remained unclear because of the combined analysis with chronic low back pain.

Yoga is clearly supported as an effective complementary treatment for chronic low back pain. Yoga to manage chronic pain from other conditions is supported in general, but it remains unclear which pain syndromes are likely to result in significant sustained improved pain outcomes. Across all pain syndromes, including chronic low back pain, further research is needed to distinguish the types of yoga that are most effective for specific pain syndromes. Bussing et al. (2012) point out the need to also disentangle the main effects for physical activity, lifestyle change, and meditation from yoga treatments. As with other complementary pain treatments, dose and treatment duration must also be empirically clarified. Clearly linking the component main effects and the specific yoga technique with the pain syndrome could provide information about the underlying mechanisms of the pain syndrome and yoga as a pain treatment.

Mindfulness Meditation

Mindfulness meditation involves focus on the interaction among cognition, physical sensations, and behavioral responses. Although many different types of mindfulness mediation exist, most share four common components that involve use of a: space with minimal distraction to practice the meditation; physically comfortable position (e.g., sitting); specific word, phrase, visual cue, or sensation as the focus for all attention; and nonjudgmental accepting attitude (NCCIH, 2018g). The majority of mindfulness meditation interventions tested with randomized clinical trials involve 8-week programs. Meta-analysis results of four RCTs supported that mindfulness when compared to attention control conditions produced a significant small pain reduction (effect size = 0.33, CI = 0.03-0.62), in which pain decreased by 5% to 31%. Mindfulness meditation when compared to other pain treatments produced no significant differences, however (Goyal et al., 2014). A second larger meta-analysis of 25 studies with high heterogeneity and less than half the studies rated as good quality supported a similar small pain reduction effect (SMD = 0.32, CI = 0.09-0.54) from mindfulness for chronic fibromyalgia, back, arthritis, headache, and irritable bowel syndrome pain (Hilton et al., 2017).

Further evidence from a rigorous RCT supports the use of mindfulness mediation for chronic back pain. Mindfulness meditation that included meditation, body scanning, and yoga classes for 2 hours each week for 8 weeks, along with mindfulness meditation at home, resulted in a clinically meaningful and statistically significant pain reduction, defined as greater than or equal to 30%, with a mean pain reduction of 48.5% (CI = 40.3%-58.3%) at 52 weeks. Pain intensity decreased by 1.42 (CI = −1.72 to −1.12) on the 0 to 10 numeric rating scale, and bothersome pain decreased by −1.95 (CI = −2.32 to −1.59), both significantly different from usual care, but not significantly different from cognitive behavioral therapy. Most importantly, the effects were sustained over a significant period of time, from 26 to 52 weeks (Cherkin et al., 2016).

Jyoti meditation significantly reduced chronic neck pain from baseline to 8 weeks of treatment for people with chronic neck pain, and did so significantly more than exercise, with a moderate effect size of 0.58. Chronic neck pain at motion was not significantly reduced, however (Jeitler et al., 2015).

Feasible and efficacious use of mindfulness meditation has some support for treating acute pain during hospitalization. A rigorous 3-arm RCT compared a 15-minute mindfulness intervention, hypnosis intervention, and education intervention. Immediately after the brief intervention, pain intensity was reduced by 30% or more for 27% of people in the mindfulness group, 39% in the hypnosis group, and only 15% in the education group. Mindfulness was no more efficacious than hypnosis but was more efficacious than no treatment (education). Mean pain intensity across the mindfulness group remained moderate, however (Garland et al., 2017).

▎Music

Music has been examined extensively as a treatment to reduce pain through either music medicine or music therapy. Music medicine consists of listening to prerecorded music with minimal support required from a healthcare professional. Music medicine is the type of music intervention tested and used most frequently. Music therapy involves more extensive and individually tailored use of music and is administered by a trained therapist (Dileo & Bradt, 2005). In the largest meta-analysis to date for the effect of music on pain outcomes, Lee (2016) analyzed 76 RCTs with $n = 6430$ participants and found that music medicine had a large effect on pain reduction, SMD $= -1.13$ (CI $= -1.44$ to -0.82); however, high heterogeneity among the RCTs ($I^2 = 95\%$) makes the findings difficult to interpret. Analysis of RCTs testing only music therapy provides clearer evidence. Meta-analysis of nine RCTs supported that music therapy reduced pain (SMD -1.50, CI $= -2.09$ to -0.91), with heterogeneity closer to an acceptable level ($I^2 = 58\%$). Meta-analysis of five RCTs of music therapy for chronic pain reduction continued to support a similar and significant effect (SMD -1.42, CI $= -1.99$ to -0.84, $I^2 = 48\%$) (Lee, 2016). Meta-analysis of 14 RCTs testing music medicine also supported a moderate effect for chronic pain reduction (SMD $= -0.60$, CI $= -0.72$ to -0.48, $I^2 = 60\%$) (Garza-Villarreal, Pando, Vuust, & Parsons, 2017). Meta-analysis of 21 music medicine RCTs testing the effect of acute pain reduction during endoscopy supported significant pain reduction from music (weighted mean difference -1.53, CI -2.53 to -0.53). The effect of music on pain during bronchoscopy and colposcopy was not significant, however (Wang et al., 2014). Meta-analysis of eight RCTs testing music therapy in adults supported a significant effect for pain reduction (SMD -1.26, CI $= -1.71$ to $-.81$, $I^2 = 26\%$) (Lee, 2016). Allowing people to select the music resulted in greater pain reduction (SMD $= -0.81$, CI $= -1.02$ to -0.59) (Garza-Villarreal et al., 2017). Music as a therapy or a simple intervention is a helpful adjunct for managing both acute and chronic pain.

Summary

Research supports each of the six reviewed complementary pain treatments (acupuncture, massage, tai chi, yoga, mindfulness, and music) as efficacious for at least one pain condition in adults. Table 8-1 summarizes the complementary pain treatments supported as efficacious for specific pain conditions. Chronic pain conditions

TABLE 8-1. Efficacious Complementary Pain Treatments for Specific Pain Conditions

Pain Condition	Acupuncture	Massage	Tai Chi	Yoga	Mindfulness	Music
Chronic low back	+			+	+	
Headache/migraine	+				+	
Osteoarthritis	+*		+*		+	
Cancer	+	+				
Fibromyalgia					+	
Irritable bowel syndrome					+	
Dysmenorrhea	+					
Chronic neck						+

TABLE **8-1**. Efficacious Complementary Pain Treatments for Specific Pain Conditions (*continued*)

Pain Condition	Acupuncture	Massage	Tai Chi	Yoga	Mindfulness	Music
Aromatase inhibitor–induced arthralgia	+					
Chronic (nonspecific)						+
Fracture	+					
Acute back					+	
Postsurgical	+	+				+
Acute (inpatient)					+	

+, Research supports the pain treatment for the pain condition.
*Research supports for knee osteoarthritis.

are listed first followed by acute pain conditions. Acupuncture and mindfulness each provide some pain relief across eight pain conditions, with three of the most common chronic pain conditions, chronic low back pain, headaches/migraines and osteoarthritis pain, responsive to both treatments. Some pain conditions respond to multiple complementary pain treatments. For example, chronic low back pain can be reduced with acupuncture, yoga, and mindfulness. Postsurgical pain can be reduced by acupuncture, massage, and music. Recent reviews also concluded that acupuncture (Chou et al., 2017; Nahin et al., 2016), tai chi (Nahin et al., 2016), and yoga and mindfulness (Chou et al., 2017) reduce chronic low back pain and that acupuncture and tai chi reduce osteoarthritis knee pain (Nahin et al., 2016).

Method issues continue to plague research efforts in complementary pain treatments and therefore need to be addressed. Complementary pain research would advance more rapidly with use of common pain outcome measures, standardized protocols for the specific complementary treatments, larger sample sizes, and more rigorous control of bias. The high heterogeneity frequently found in the meta-analyses might be further reduced by inclusion of moderators and/or mediators relevant to the complementary treatment and pain condition. As with any therapeutic intervention, treatment dose and length of effect need to be more clearly substantiated to better guide practitioners and people in pain.

Research evidence supports that for adults, specific complementary treatments reduce pain for some specific conditions. Underlying pain mechanisms might be further elucidated by examining underlying complementary treatment mechanisms that relieve pain for specific conditions. Findings would inform more precise pain treatments and result in greater pain relief. Practitioner guidance to match appropriate complementary pain treatments with specific pain conditions remains crucial for optimal pain self-management in adults suffering from acute and chronic pain.

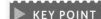 **KEY POINT**

Practitioner guidance to match appropriate complementary pain treatments with specific pain conditions remains crucial for optimal pain self-management in adults suffering from acute and chronic pain.

REFERENCES

Boiter, M., Gelinas, C., Richard-Lalonde, M., & Thombs, B. (2017). The effect of massage on acute postoperative pain in critically and acutely ill adults post-thoracic surgery: Systematic review and meta-analysis of randomized controlled trials. *Heart & Lung, 46*, 339–346.

Boyd, C., Crawford, C., Paat, C., Price, A., Xenakis, L., & Zhang, W. (2016a). The impact of massage therapy on function in pain populations—A systematic review and meta-analysis of randomized controlled trials: Part III, surgical pain populations. *Pain Medicine, 17*, 1757–1772. doi:10.1093/pm/pnw/101

Boyd, C., Crawford, C., Paat, C., Price, A., Xenakis, L., & Zhang, W. (2016b). The impact of massage therapy on function in pain populations—A systematic review and meta-analysis of randomized controlled trials: Part II, cancer pain populations. *Pain Medicine, 17*, 1553–1568. doi:10.1093/pm/pnw/100

Bussing, A., Ostermann, T., Ludtke, R., & Michalsen, A. (2012). Effects of yoga interventions on pain and pain-associated disability: A meta-analysis. *The Journal of Pain, 13*, 1–9. doi:10.1016/j.jpain.2011.10.001

Chen, L., Lin, C., Huang, T., Kuan, Y., Huang, Y., Chen, H., . . . Tam., K. (2017). Effect of acupuncture on aromatase inhibitor-induced arthralgia in patients with breast cancer: A meta-analysis of randomized controlled trials. *The Breast, 33*, 132–138. doi:10.1016/j .breast.2017.03.015

Cherkin, D., Sherman, K., Balderson, B., Cook, A., Anderson, M., Hawkes, R., . . . Turner, J. (2016). Effect of mindfulness-based stress reduction vs cognitive behavioral therapy or usual care on back pain and functional limitations in adults with chronic low back pain a randomized clinical trial. *Journal of the American Medical Association, 315*, 1240–1249. doi:10.1001/jama.2016.2323

Chiu, H., Hsieh, Y., & Tsai, P. (2016). Systematic review and meta-analysis of acupuncture to reduce cancer-related pain. *European Journal of Cancer Care, 26*, e12457. doi:10.1111/ ecc.12457

Cho, Y., Kim, C., Heo, K., Lee, M., Ha, I., Son, D., . . . Shin, B. (2015). Acupuncture for acute postoperative pain after back surgery: A systematic review and meta-analysis of randomized controlled trials. *Pain Practice, 15*, 279–291. doi:10.1111/papr.12208

Chou, R., Deyo, R., Friedly, J., Skelly, A., Hashimoto, R., Weimer, M., . . . Brodt, E. (2017). Nonpharmacological therapies for low back pain: A systematic review for an American College of Physicians Clinical Practice Guideline. *Annuals of Internal Medicine, 166*, 493–505. doi:10.7326/M16-2459

Clarke, T., Black, L., Stussman, B., Barnes, P., & Nahin, R. (2015). Trends in the use of complementary health approaches among adults: United States, 2002–2012. *National Health Statistics Reports, 10*, 1–16.

Crawford, C., Boyd, C., Paat, C., Price, A., Xenakis, L., Yang, E., & Zhang, W. (2016). The Impact of massage therapy on function in pain populations—A systematic review and meta-analysis of randomized controlled trials: Part I, patients experiencing pain in the general population. *Pain Medicine, 17*, 1353–1375. doi:10.1093/pm/pnw099

Dileo, C., & Bradt, J. (2005). *Medical music therapy: A meta-analysis & agenda for future research*. Cherry Hill, NJ: Jeffery Books.

Garland, E., Baker, A., Larsen, P., Riquino, M., Priddy, S., Thomas, E., . . . Nakamura, Y. (2017). Randomized controlled trial of brief mindfulness training and hypnotic suggestion for acute pain relief in the hospital setting. *Journal of General Internal Medicine, 32*, 1106–1113. doi:10.1007/s11606-017-4116-9

Garza-Villarreal, E., Pando, V., Vuust, P., & Parsons, C. (2017). Music-induced analgesia in chronic pain conditions: A systematic review and meta-analysis. *Pain Physician, 20*, 597–610.

Goyal, M., Singh, S., Sibinga, E., Gould, N., Rowland-Seymour, A., Sharma, R., . . . Haythorn-waite, J. (2014). Meditation programs for psychological stress and well-being: A systematic review and meta-analysis. *Journal of the American Medical Association Internal Medicine, 174,* 357–368. doi:10.1001/jamainternmed.2013.13018

Hall, A., Copsey, B., Richmond, H., Thompson, J., Ferreira, M., Latimer, J., & Maher, C. (2017). Effectiveness of tai chi for chronic musculoskeletal pain conditions: Updated systematic review and meta-analysis. *Physical Therapy, 97,* 227–238.

Hilton, L., Hempel, S., Ewing, B., Apaydin, E., Xenakis, L., Newberry, S., . . . Maglione, M. (2017). Mindfulness meditation for chronic pain: Systematic review and meta-analysis. *Annals of Behavioral Medicine, 51,* 199–213. doi:10.1007/s12160-016-9844-2

Holtzman, S., & Beggs, R. (2013). Yoga for chronic low back pain: A meta-analysis of randomized controlled trials. *Pain Research & Management, 18,* 267–272.

Jan, A., Aldridge, E., Rogers, I., Visser, E., Bulsara, M., & Niemtzow, R. (2017). Review article: Does acupuncture have a role in providing analgesia in the emergency setting? A systematic review and meta-analysis. *Emergency Medicine Australasia, 29,* 490–498. doi:10.1111/1742-6723.12832

Jeitler, M., Brunnhuber, S., Meier, L., Ludtke, R., Bussing, A., Kessler, C., & Michaelsen, A. (2015). Effectiveness of Jyoti medication for patients with chronic neck pain and psychological distress—A randomized controlled clinical trial. *The Journal of Pain, 16,* 77–86. doi:10.1016/j.jpain.2014.10.009

Kong, L., Lauche, R., Klose, P., Bu, J., Yang, X., Guo, C., . . . Cheng, Y. (2016). Tai chi for chronic pain conditions: A systematic review and meta-analysis of randomized controlled trials. *Scientific Reports, 6,* 25325. doi:10.1038/srep25325

Lam, M., Galvin, R., & Curry, P. (2013). Effectiveness of acupuncture for nonspecific chronic low back pain. *Spine, 38,* 2124–2138. doi:10.1097/01.brs.0000435025.65564.b7

Law, D., McDonough, S., Bleakley, C., Baxter, G., & Tumilty, S. (2015). Laser acupuncture for treating musculoskeletal pain: A systematic review with meta-analysis. *Journal of Acupuncture and Meridian Studies, 8,* 2–16. doi:10.1016/j.jams.2014.06.015

Lee, J. (2016). The effect of music on pain. *Journal of Music Therapy, 53,* 430–477. doi:10.1093/jmt/thw012

Lee, S., Kim, J., Yeo, S., Kim, S. & Lim, S. (2015). Meta-analysis of massage therapy on cancer pain. *Integrative Cancer Therapies, 14,* 297–304. doi:10.1177/1534735415572885

Manyanga, T., Froese, M., Zarychanski, R., Abou-Setta, A., Friesen, C., Tennenhouse, M., & Shay, B. (2014). Pain management with acupuncture in osteoarthritis: A systematic review and meta-analysis. *BMC Complementary & Alternative Medicine, 14,* 312.

Nahin, R., Boineau, R., Khalsa, P., Stussman, B., & Weber, W. (2016). Evidence-based evaluation of complementary health approaches for pain management in the United States. *Mayo Clinical Proceedings, 91,* 1292–1306. doi:10.1016/j.mayocp.2016.06.007

Nahin, R., Stussman, B., & Herman, P. (2015). Out-of-pocket expenditures on complementary health approaches associated with painful health conditions in a nationally representative adult sample. *The Journal of Pain, 16,* 1147–1162. doi:10.1016/j.jpain.2015.07.013

National Center for Complementary and Integrative Health. (2018a). *Complementary, alternative, or integrative health: What's in a name?* Retrieved from https://nccih.nih.gov/health/integrative-health#hed1

National Center for Complementary and Integrative Health. (2018b). *Chiropractic.* Retrieved from https://nccih.nih.gov/health/chiropractic/introduction.htm

National Center for Complementary and Integrative Health. (2018c). *Spinal manipulation for low-back pain.* Retrieved from https://nccih.nih.gov/health/pain/spinemanipulation.htm

National Center for Complementary and Integrative Health. (2018d). *Acupuncture.* https://nccih.nih.gov/health/acupuncture

National Center for Complementary and Integrative Health. (2018e). *Spotlight on a modality: Tai chi*. Retrieved from https://nccih.nih.gov/health/providers/digest/taichi

National Center for Complementary and Integrative Health. (2018f). *Yoga: What you need to know*. Retrieved from https://nccih.nih.gov/health/yoga/introduction.htm

National Center for Complementary and Integrative Health. (2018g). *Meditation: In depth*. Retrieved from https://nccih.nih.gov/health/meditation/overview.htm#hed2

Wang, M., Zhang, L., Zhang, X., Zhang, Y., Dong, X., & Zhang Y. C. (2014). Effect of music in endoscopy procedures: Systematic review and meta-analysis of randomized controlled trials. *Pain Medicine, 15*, 1786–1794.

Ward, L., Stebbings, S., Cherkin, D., & Baxter, G. (2013). Yoga for functional ability, pain and psychosocial outcomes in musculoskeletal conditions: A systematic review and meta-analysis. *Musculoskeletal Care, 11*, 203–217. doi:10.1002/msc.1042

Woo, H., Ji, H., Pak, Y., Lee, H., Heo, S., Lee, J., & Park, K. (2018). The efficacy and safety of acupuncture in women with primary dysmenorrhea. *Medicine, 97*, e11007. doi:10.1097/MD.0000000000011007

CHAPTER 9

INTERVENTIONAL PAIN MANAGEMENT

Joseph Walker, Miguel Ernesto Velez, and Moorice Caparó

Introduction

Interventional pain treatment options are an important component in the multi-modal approach for pain management. Interventional pain options treat the symptom of pain, potentially allowing the individual to participate in other available treatment options such as physical therapy and cognitive behavioral therapy. This reduction in pain level can improve functional outcomes. Many interventional treatments are available for the patient, and the indications for them vary as well. Selecting the correct interventional procedure, whether for spinal pain, neuropathic pain, orthopedic pain, head/neck pain, or malignant pain, can help the progression of a patient's healing. The goal of this chapter is to give an organized overview of the various interventional pain treatment modalities that are available for a patient's plan of care.

KEY POINT

Interventional pain management techniques play an essential part in a multidisciplinary approach to relieve pain.

Spinal Pain Interventions

Spinal pain encompasses diagnoses that involve the structural components of the cervical, thoracic, lumbar, or sacrum. The potential treatment targets within the spinal column include the spinal nerve roots, the spinal articular structures, and even the spinal cord itself.

KEY POINT

Although mechanisms are not completely understood, improvement in radicular pain after an epidural steroid injection may be attributed to attenuation of inflammatory mediators and neuronal hyperexcitability at the level of the spinal root, dorsal ganglia, or dorsal horn (Leak, 2006).

Epidural Steroid Injections

Introduction

Epidural steroid injections have been a mainstay of both subacute and chronic back pain management for many years. The procedure is used to treat radicular pain originating from the cervical, thoracic, or lumbar regions of the spine. There are many underlying causes of radicular pain. The most common include: (1) nerve root compression from disk herniation, (2) spondylosis, (3) spinal stenosis, or (4) postlaminectomy pain syndrome (Boswell et al., 2007).

Epidural steroid injections can help maintain conservative treatment, predict surgical outcome, reduce opioid use, and improve return to work.

Clinical Features

Although a patient's presentation may vary, radicular symptoms are generally described as sharp, burning, or shooting sensation that radiates down an extremity. This radiating referral pattern typically follows a specific dermatomal distribution. Paresthesia may also be reported. Patient may also complain of motor weakness when performing certain functions such as dorsiflexion (L4-L5), hip flexion (L2-L4), and plantar flexion (S1). Patients with spinal stenosis will have complaints because of symptoms of neurogenic claudication. This includes (1) pain that is worse after standing and walking followed by pain relief soon after sitting down and (2) pain while going downstairs compared to going up as stenosis and pain are reduced with spine flexion (Friedrich & Harrast, 2010). For all patients presenting with radicular pain, a history of bowel and bladder function must be obtained as impaired function may point toward spinal cord compression needing neurosurgical consultation. Severe and/or rapidly progressing neurologic symptoms should also warrant further workup and possible neurosurgical evaluation (Allegri et al., 2016).

Physical examination findings

Careful physical examination of the myotome (motor strength), dermatome (sensation), and deep tendon reflexes of the various spinal segments must be performed in order to help clinically localize the spinal level of involvement. Examples of lumbar myotomal weakness include: weakness with plantar flexor or hip extension for an S1 root involvement, weakness with foot eversion or hip abduction for L5 root involvement, or weakness with ankle dorsiflexion or knee extension for L4 root involvement. Within a specific dermatomal distribution, the patient may exhibit loss of sensation to light touch, allodynia with the pinch-roll test, or hyperalgesia with pinprick test. Neural tension maneuvers on physical examination, such as the Spurling's maneuver for the cervical spine and supine straight leg raise for the lumbar spine, may help localize nerve root impingement because of disk herniation. These physical examination tests also screen for spinal cord involvement in red flag situations such as myelopathy or central cord syndrome. Signs of spinal cord involvement include frank hyperreflexia, clonus, or absent/pathologic reflexes (Hoffman or Babinski signs) (Allegri et al., 2016).

Interventional procedure type

 KEY POINT

Injection into the epidural space via transforaminal, interlaminar, or caudal approach in the cervical, thoracic, or lumbar regions of the spine.

Brief description of procedure

The procedure consists of placing steroid medication to the epidural space. The epidural space is located between the dura and the spinal canal. The dura is the outermost covering of spinal cord. Both the epidural injection procedure approach and the selected spinal level to inject are individualized. These two variables depend on (1) patient presentation, (2) findings on imaging, (3) practice preference, (4) prior surgery, and (5) previous response to other epidural injections (Patel, Wasserman, & Imani, 2015).

▶ *Transforaminal Approach* (Figure 9-1)—The target for this approach is the space between each vertebra where the nerve exits the spinal canal, called the neural foramina. The neural foramina are located more laterally. This approach places the medication more anteriorly in the epidural space and closely targets the specific nerve root that exits at that level on that side.

▶ *Interlaminar Approach* (Figures 9-2 and 9-3)—The target for this approach is the space between the lamina of subsequent vertebrae. The space is located posteriorly just slightly off midline. This approach places the medication more in the posterior aspect of the epidural space.

▶ *Caudal Approach* (Figure 9-4)—The target for this approach is the sacral hiatus that is located at the distal part of the sacrum and may access the epidural space. This approach places the medication in the caudal aspect of the spinal column, targeting more of the lower lumbar and sacral roots. This technique can be useful in the postsurgical spine as the transforaminal and interlaminar space may be altered.

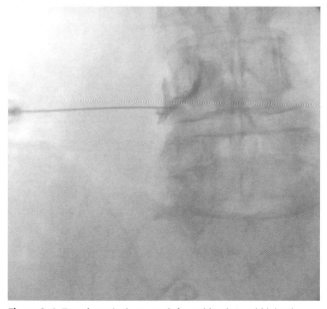

Figure 9–1. Transforaminal approach for epidural steroid injection.

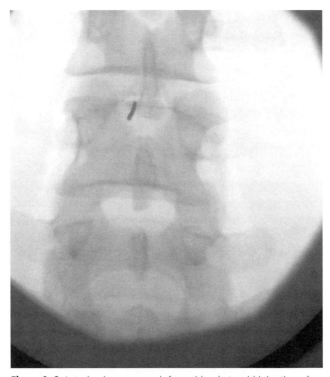

Figure 9−2. Interlaminar approach for epidural steroid injection of the lumbar spine.

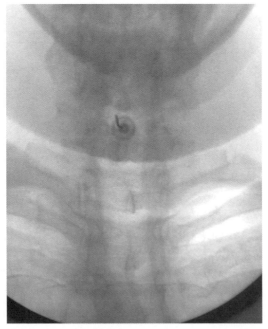

Figure 9−3. Interlaminar approach for epidural steroid injection of the cervical spine.

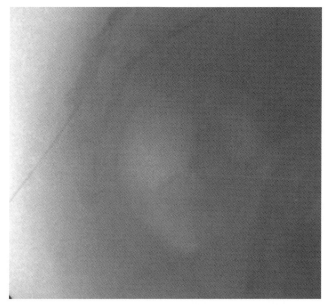

Figure 9–4. Caudal approach for epidural steroid injection.

Contraindications

The contraindications for the procedure include active systemic infection or infection of the overlying skin, anticoagulation or problems with coagulation, hypersensitivity to steroids, contrast dye, anesthetic medications, and local malignancy. Special considerations should be had in patients with uncontrolled diabetes, heart failure, and pregnancy (Patel & Upadhyayula, 2018).

Risk/potential adverse effects

Direct injection into the nerve root or even spinal cord can result in acute spinal cord injury. Needle puncture and injection into the intervertebral disk may predispose to diskitis (Patel, Wasserman, & Imani, 2015). Epidural hematomas may result from injury to the vascular bundle as it enters the neural foramina. Dural tears, vasovagal syncope, and systemic corticosteroid side effects have also been seen in practice (Friedrich & Harrast, 2010).

Imaging modalities used to perform procedure

Epidural steroid injections were originally done without any image guidance. This lack of visual confirmation resulted in inaccurate needle placement in up to 30% of cases. This was even in the hands of experienced clinicians (Patel, Wasserman, & Imani, 2015).

Fluoroscopy is by far more common as it involves less radiation overall. Ultrasound guidance has been used for needle placement as well.

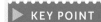
KEY POINT

Fluoroscopic or computed tomography (CT) guidance is now the standard of care that greatly improves procedure accuracy and overall safety.

Type of medications used

A combination of steroid and local anesthetic is used within the injectate. There is no consensus in the dosage or type of corticosteroid used. Radiopaque water-soluble contrast is used to confirm needle placement. Contrast material is used to assist with avoidance of intravascular injection of the steroid injectate (Patel, Wasserman, & Imani, 2015).

Sedations used

Sedation is not typically used for this procedure.

Length of time for the procedure

Five to 10 minutes.

Expected postprocedural care

Typical postprocedural restrictions/limitations include: (1) avoidance of driving, (2) avoidance of strenuous activity following procedure, and (3) avoidance of submerging the injection site in water. The patient should be closely monitored for worsening of pain, signs of infection, or systemic corticosteroid side effects. Immediate medical help should be sought if patient experiences sudden-onset weakness or loss of bowel/bladder function following procedure.

Frequency of having this procedure

There is no consensus on timing and frequency of epidural steroid injections. Some international interventional spine societies recommend no more than four injections in a 6-month period.

Gauging the patient's response to prior injection is essential to determine if another injection is warranted (Friedrich & Harrast, 2010).

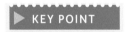
KEY POINT

The common practice to limit no more than three to four epidural injections per year is to decrease the risk of systemic steroid side effects.

Ways of documentation of efficacy

Documentation of treatment outcome can be done via (1) the numeric rating scale and (2) the visual analog scale at different time intervals during treatment.

Zygapophyseal Joint Interventions

Introduction

The zygapophyseal, or facet, joints are a common cause of chronic back and neck pain. Over time, the zygapophyseal joints undergo osteoarthritic degenerative changes. These degenerative joint changes when combined with degenerative disk changes are collectively called spondylosis. Spondylosis accounts for 10% to 50% of all chronic lower back pain cases (Schwarzer et al., 1994).

The superior articular processes of the lower vertebrae articulate with the inferior articular processes of the vertebrae above (Gellhorn, Katz, & Suri, 2013).

Facet joints are innervated by the medial branches of the dorsal primary rami of the spinal nerves.

Clinical features

The axial pain may be unilateral or bilateral. Zygapophyseal joint–mediated pain may also radiate into the upper and lower extremities. This type of pain may present with localized referred patterns to the occiput, posterior scapular/shoulder, buttocks, or the thighs (Gellhorn, Katz, & Suri, 2013).

Physical examination findings

Specific physical examination findings for facet joint–mediated pain are worsening pain with extension, pain with extension–rotation also known as Kemp's test, and palpatory tenderness along facet joint line.

Interventional procedure type

The injection is either intraarticular into the facet joint or onto the medial branch nerve. The rhizotomy targets the medial branch nerve.

Brief description of procedure

A radiofrequency ablation (RFA) is also known as facet joint neurotomy or rhizotomy. RFA is typically performed after the medial branch block or facet joint injection. This procedure is primarily therapeutic and can provide pain relief for as long as 6 to 12 months. While the patient is in the prone position, the skin is cleaned and draped in a sterile fashion. The target levels are determined based on anatomic landmarks under fluoroscopy.

▶ For facet joint injections (Figures 9-5 and 9-6): After administering local anesthetic superficially, the spinal needle is guided intraarticularly into the zygapophyseal joint. A combination of anesthetic and steroid is then administered. The facet joint injection is a therapeutic procedure.

▶ For medial branch block: After administering local anesthetic superficially, the spinal needle is guided to the location of the medial branch nerve. The medial branch nerve is found at the junction of the superior articular process and transverse process (for thoracic and lumbar) or at the lateral masses (for cervical). The zygapophyseal joint is dually innervated and as such two medial branches need to be injected for a single zygapophyseal joint. Anesthetic and/or steroid is then administered. The medial branch block is a diagnostic procedure.

> ▶ **KEY POINT**
>
> The zygapophyseal joints are paired diarthrodial joints located in the posterior aspect of the vertebral column and connect the adjacent vertebrae.

> ▶ **KEY POINT**
>
> Zygapophyseal joint–mediated pain typically presents as localized neck, midback, or low back pain.

> ▶ **KEY POINT**
>
> The physical examination findings can be very nonspecific, and diagnosis is usually confirmed after a facet joint injection or a medial branch block.

> ▶ **KEY POINT**
>
> A medial branch block injection or an intraarticular facet joint injection with an anesthetic can be both therapeutic and diagnostic as they can confirm the etiology of the pain as from the facet joints.

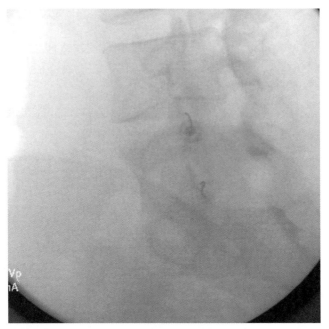

Figure 9-5. Facet joint injection of the lumbar spine.

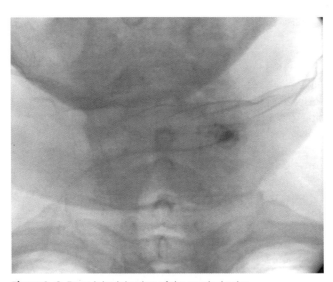

Figure 9-6. Facet joint injection of the cervical spine.

▶ For RFA: After administering local anesthetic, a radiofrequency probe is guided to the location of the medial branch nerve (Gadsen, 2013). The medial branch nerve is found at the junction of the superior articular process and transverse process (for thoracic and lumbar) or at the lateral masses (for cervical). Sensory and motor stimulation is done to confirm that the ventral ramus or spinal nerves are not being ablated. Ablation is then performed with the radiofrequency generator at 80°C to 85°C for 90 seconds (Manchikanti et al., 2003). Once again, the zygapophyseal joint is dually innervated and as such the ablation is performed at a minimum of two medial branches to influence a single zygapophyseal joint. RFA is a therapeutic procedure.

Contraindications

As with other spine injection procedures, the contraindications for the procedure include active infections, allergies, active pregnancy, inability to come off anticoagulation, and inability to position for the procedure.

Risk/potential adverse effects

As with other spinal injections, the complications are usually related to needle placement and drug administration. The complications include dural puncture, spinal cord injury, infection, intravascular injection, spinal anesthesia, chemical meningitis, neural trauma, pneumothorax, and hematoma formation. Vertebral artery injury is more common with cervical intraarticular injections (Manchikanti et al., 2003). Most problems, such as local swelling, pain at the site of the needle insertion, and pain in the low back, are typically self-limited.

Imaging modalities used to perform procedure

The procedure is most commonly performed under fluoroscopic guidance. Ultrasound has been utilized also for visualization of needle/radiofrequency probe placement. Other less commonly used imaging modalities include CT and magnetic resonance imaging (MRI) (Manchikanti et al., 2015).

Type of medications used

Facet joint injections and RFA both typically use local anesthetics such as lidocaine or bupivacaine for superficial infiltration. Facet joint injections use a steroid as the primary injectate into the joint. Medial branch blocks use either a short-acting or a long-acting local anesthetic alone for the injection of the medial branch nerve. During the RFA procedure, some providers may inject steroid at the nerve in addition to the rhizotomy, although evidence of improved pain relief is limited.

Sedations used

These procedures are usually without sedation, although this may vary depending on the patient or provider. If sedation is utilized, midazolam or fentanyl is typically used. Studies have shown that administration of sedation can be a confounding factor in the diagnosis of facet joint–mediated pain with medial branch block (Manchikanti et al., 2004, 2016).

Length of time for the procedure

Five to 30 minutes. Length of time for the procedure depends on the provider skillset and the number of levels being done.

Expected postprocedural care

Patients are typically advised to rest for the remainder of the day, to limit heavy lifting and to avoid strenuous activity. If sedation is administered, the patient is to avoid driving and operating heavy machinery for the remainder of the day after the procedure.

Frequency of having this procedure

The specific frequency of the treatments performed may vary depending on the effect of the procedure and provider preference.

Ways of documentation of efficacy

Documentation of treatment outcome can be done via (1) numeric rating scale, (2) visual analog scale, (3) functional status, and (4) health-related quality of life scale (EuroQual-5 dimensions; EQ5D) (Manchikanti et al., 2015).

> ▶ **KEY POINT**
>
> Medial branch block and facet joint injections are done to confirm diagnosis of facet joint–mediated pain. Once the diagnosis has been established, RFA can be performed every 6 to 12 months.

Sacroiliac Joint Injections

Introduction

The sacroiliac joint is a true synovial joint between the sacrum and the ilium, and although it is a relatively immobile joint, it is involved in transferring weight from the trunk to the lower extremities (Raj & Dulebohn, 2017). Pain and dysfunction can be attributed to abnormal movement or misalignment, trauma, inflammation, and pregnancy (Forst, Wheeler, Fortin, & Vilensky, 2006).

> ▶ **KEY POINT**
>
> The patient complains of unilateral lower back pain, which typically radiates into buttock, posterior leg, or posterolateral leg.

Clinical features

The radiating pain does not usually extend below the knee. Groin pain is another referral pattern in a subset of patients (Jung et al., 2007).

Physical examination findings

The patient may point directly to the area within 1 cm of the posterior superior iliac crest (Fortin's finger test). Pain can be reproduced by placing direct stress on the sacroiliac joint. This can be done via the sacroiliac joint distraction maneuver, sacral thigh thrusts in supine position, or with compression at the lateral hip while patient is side lying. Patrick's test also known as FABER (Flexion, Abduction, and External Rotation) test has been reported as having highest positivity in patients with confirmed sacroiliac joint pathology (Telli et al., 2018). Other provocative tests include Gaenslen's test in which the patient is placed at the edge of the examination table in supine position, with one hip maximally extended and the opposite hip maximally flexed.

> ▶ **KEY POINT**
>
> On physical examination of the sacroiliac joint, no single physical examination maneuver is used as the gold standard diagnostic test (Szadek et al., 2008). A combination of tests may have a higher sensitivity and specificity.

Interventional procedure type

The injection is intraarticular into the sacroiliac joint.

Brief description of procedure

Patient is placed prone. The fluoroscopy machine is positioned over distal one third to one fifth of sacroiliac joint. The spinal needle is guided toward posterior aspect of joint (Figure 9-7). Needle depth can be confirmed with an oblique or lateral fluoroscopic view. Once the intraarticular joint space is reached, needle placement is confirmed with radiopaque contrast. Approximately 1 to 3 mL of injectate, a combination of steroid and local anesthetic, is then injected into the joint (Patel, Wasserman, & Imani, 2015).

Contraindications

The contraindications for the procedure include systemic or local active infections, active pregnancy, uncontrolled diabetes, malignancy, allergies to injectate.

Risk/potential adverse effects

The complications are usually related infection, spread of medication to adjacent tissue, bleeding, bruising, and pain at injection site.

Imaging modalities used to perform procedure

Sacroiliac joint injections may be done without image guidance. This, however, increases the risk of injury to surrounding tissue given the deep nature of the sacroiliac

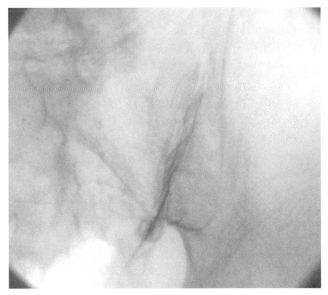

Figure 9-7. Sacroiliac joint injection.

joint (Pang, Mahajan, & Fishmann, 2005). Fluoroscopic guidance is preferred over CT guidance because of concern for increased radiation exposure and overall expense. Low-dose CT protocols may decrease radiation exposure to that of pulsed fluoroscopy (Artner, Cakir, Reichel, & Lattig, 2012). Ultrasound is also an emerging way for needle guidance.

Type of medications used

An anesthetic such a lidocaine or bupivacaine is usually mixed with a corticosteroid for longer term effects. Viscosupplementation with hyaluronic acid may be used (Srejic, Calvillo, & Kabakibou, 1999).

Sedations used

Sedation is not used during this procedure.

Length of time for the procedure

Five to 10 minutes.

Expected postprocedural care

Patients are typically advised to avoid submerging injection site in water and to avoid strenuous activity immediately following procedure (Dussault, Kaplan, & Anderson, 2000).

Frequency of having this procedure

The number of procedures yearly varies but typically numbers about three in a 12-month period. Frequency will depend on patient's response to treatment and physician's preference.

Ways of documentation of efficacy

Documentation of treatment outcome can be done via (1) visual analog scale and (2) numeric pain rating scale (Scholten, Patel, Christos, & Singh, 2015).

▌Spinal Cord Stimulation

Introduction

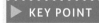

KEY POINT

The medical literature supports positive results in neuropathic and vascular insufficiency pain (Huber & Vaglienti, 2000; Manchikanti et al., 2003).

Used to treat chronic and intractable pain, spinal cord stimulation (SCS) is accomplished via an implantable subcutaneous device.

Common indications for SCS include complex regional pain syndrome (CRPS) (Types I and II), failed back surgery syndrome (FBSS), peripheral vascular disease, visceral pain (such as intractable angina), and peripheral neuropathy (Mekhail et al., 2011; Latif, Nedeljkovic, & Stevenson, 2001). CRPS (Types I and II) and FBSS account for 82% of the cases where SCS is utilized.

Clinical features

The two most common indications for SCS are briefly reviewed here.

- ▶ Complex Regional Pain Syndrome: CRPS (Types I and II) is neuropathic/sympathetically mediated pain syndrome. CRPS Type I presents without a known nerve damage, whereas Type II presents with known nerve damage. Patients typically report hyperesthesia, allodynia, temperature changes, skin color changes, decreased range of motion, decreased strength, trophic changes (such as changes in hair, nail, or skin), and edema (Freedman et al., 2014).
- ▶ Failed back surgery syndrome: FBSS encompasses a constellation of conditions describing recurring low back pain, with or without neuropathic pain, following one or more spine surgeries. It is important to (1) assess the pain characteristics, (2) exclude other serious diagnoses, and (3) compare to the patient's presurgical pain (Chan & Peng, 2011).

Physical examination findings

- ▶ CRPS: Physical examination findings may include hyperalgesia to pinprick, allodynia to pinch and roll test, temperature asymmetry, sweating changes or asymmetry, decreased range of motion, weakness, tremor, dystonia, and trophic changes (Freedman et al., 2014; Maleki et al., 2000).
- ▶ FBSS: The physical examination is similar to any comprehensive back pain examination and it should be focused and directed by the findings provided on the history (Chan & Peng, 2011).

Interventional procedure type

The SCS trial is an outpatient interventional spine procedure. The SCS permanent placement is a surgical procedure.

Brief description of procedure

Before a permanent subcutaneous device is implanted, an SCS trial lasting between 5 and 7 days is done with an external device. However, lead placement is done in a similar fashion in both cases. General anesthesia is then administered. Spinal anatomic landmarks are determined by using fluoroscopy. A needle is inserted into the epidural space. A stimulator lead is then advanced through the needle. The second lead is placed in the same fashion on the opposite side. After coverage of stimulation is confirmed, the needles are withdrawn, leaving the leads in place. If a paddle lead is used for a greater coverage area, a laminectomy may need to be done for permanent lead placement. If the lead trial is successful in terms of pain relief, functioning, and decreased analgesic medication usage, the permanent leads and device are then placed.

Contraindications

The contraindications for the procedure include infection, anticoagulation, history of cardiac device implantation, severe spondylolisthesis with stenosis, severe scoliosis, and prior spine surgery with epidural scarring (Kreis & Fischman, 2009).

Risk/potential adverse effects

The complications of this procedure include poor paresthesia coverage, lead migration or breakage, failure of electrode lead, infection, bleeding, paralysis, nerve injury, and death (Manchikanti et al., 2003).

Imaging modalities used to perform procedure

Both the SCS trial and permanent placement are done under fluoroscopic guidance.

Type of medications used

Local anesthetic such as lidocaine is typically used superficially.

Sedations used

General anesthesia is typically done for lead placement.

Length of time for the procedure

The lead insertion placement may require between 30 minutes and 1 hour. The patient may require an overnight hospital stay.

Expected postprocedural care

Recovery takes between 6 and 8 weeks. Patients should refrain from strenuous physical activity, twisting, bending, or heavy lifting (Sjm.com, 2018).

Frequency of having this procedure

After an SCS trial and permanent device placement, further procedures are typically not performed unless a revision is needed.

Ways of documentation of efficacy

Documentation of treatment outcome can be done via visual analog pain scale, Oswestry Disability Index, sickness impact profile (SIP), health-related quality of life, EQ5D, functional level, activities of daily living, analgesic use, work status, and CRPS severity score (Barolat et al., 2001; Burton, 1975; Manchikanti et al., 2003).

▌Intrathecal Drug Delivery Systems

Introduction

Intrathecal drug delivery systems are established alternatives for the management of pain and spasticity when less invasive options are not feasible or have proven ineffective.

Medication is delivered directly into the intrathecal space via subcutaneously inserted pump and catheter system. Standard practice includes a trial of the medication injected directly into intrathecal space. If it proves effective, then the patient will undergo permanent surgical implantation of pump and reservoir system (Duarte, Raphael, & Eldabe, 2016).

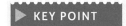

KEY POINT

Procedure is indicated for cancer and noncancer pain as well as spasticity that is refractory to other medication alternatives.

Clinical features

The typical patient who presents for intrathecal drug delivery has (1) the above-mentioned diagnoses, (2) a long-standing and complex pain history, and (3) attempted multiple treatment modalities such as oral medications and invasive procedures. The physical examination performed is specific for the presenting diagnosis. Spasticity is graded using the Modified Ashworth Scale (Duarte et al., 2011).

Interventional procedure type

The trial for the efficacy of the intrathecal drug is an outpatient interventional procedure. The implantation of the intrathecal drug delivery system is a surgical procedure. The delivery system is subcutaneously implanted and the corresponding reservoir system is placed intrathecally. Both are connected to each other via a catheter.

Brief description of procedure

Device implantation usually occurs after a successful trial of medication delivered intrathecally whereupon the patient had some sustained pain relief. The procedure consists of two incisions. The first incision is for the intrathecal catheter that is placed in the thoracolumbar area posteriorly, which is anchored to the underlying fascia. The second incision is for pump and reservoir system implantation that is typically positioned in the abdominal wall but may also be positioned in other areas. Specific pump placement will vary depending on patient preference (such as sleeping position), avoidance of bony landmarks, and other anatomic limitations. Pump system is placed at a depth of 1.5 to 2.5 cm to allow for easy access for refilling procedures. Reservoir systems will need to be refilled at least every 6 months, although they are usually refilled on a 3- to 4-month basis depending upon medication dosing. During the refilling process, the pump is accessed percutaneously via the self-sealing silicone septum that is located in the center of the anterior aspect of the pump system (Bottros & Christo, 2014).

Contraindications

Contraindications for the procedure include the following: patients who fail trial of intrathecal medication administration, patients unwilling to undergo regular pump refills, coagulopathy, systemic anticoagulation, active systemic or local infection, intracranial hypertension, spinal cord pathology with cerebrospinal fluid obstruction, significant emaciation preventing device implantation, and significant psychiatric illness (Bottros & Christo, 2014; Eldabe, Duarte, Raphael, Thomson, & Bojanic, 2015).

Risk/potential adverse effects

The potential adverse effects from this procedure are both general and specific. Generally, as with any other surgery, surgical site infection, bleeding, and bruising post-procedure can be encountered.

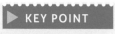

KEY POINT

Specific adverse effects for this procedure are related infusion of the medication and the status of the catheter.

Patients need to be monitored closely for signs of withdrawal and overdose of medication being used intrathecally. Symptoms of withdrawal include sudden increase in spasticity, fever, tachycardia, hallucinations, and seizures. Other device-specific complications include: catheter kinking, catheter dislodgement, delivery device failure, programming failure, and neural axial infections (epidural abscess, meningitis). Although rare, neurologic deficits have been reported from inflammatory mass development at catheter tip and neurotoxicity of medication (Knight, Brand, Mchaourab, & Veneziano, 2007).

Imaging modalities used to perform procedure

The trial and the implantation procedure is performed under fluoroscopy guidance to confirm intrathecal positioning (Duarte, Raphael, & Eldabe, 2016).

Types of medications used

The most common medications used for continuous intrathecal delivery include: (1) opioids (such as morphine and hydromorphone), (2) local anesthetics (such as bupivacaine), (3) antispasmodic medications (such as baclofen), and others such as clonidine and ziconotide (Eldabe et al., 2015).

Sedations used

The trial is done under local anesthesia. The permanent device implantation is done under sedation. The refilling process requires local anesthesia.

Length of time for the procedure

The procedural time for the intrathecal trial of medication usually is 15 to 30 minutes. The implantation of the delivery device, reservoir, and intrathecal catheter may take 1 to 4 hours. Postimplantation surgical care will likely require an overnight stay for vital sign monitoring and medication dose titration. Refilling procedure is an outpatient procedure and typically takes 15 to 30 minutes.

Expected postprocedural care

Careful monitoring is done for any signs and symptoms of complications such as medication overdose/withdrawal, infections, and cerebrospinal fluid leak. Patients must have clearly defined pathways for dealing with complications and possible adverse effects (i.e., knowing who to call or where to go if a situation were to arise). Patients are instructed to avoid hot tubs/hot showers/saunas as well as scuba diving over 10 m as changes in pressure and temperature may affect the flow rate of the medication within the system (Eldabe et al., 2015; Knight et al., 2007).

Frequency of having this procedure

Implantation is typically a one-time permanent procedure but may be removed if any complication occurs. The refilling process typically occurs once to twice a year.

Ways of documentation of efficacy

Documentation of treatment outcome can be done via (1) visual analog pain scale, (2) patient self-reported side effects, (3) Modified Ashworth Scale, and (4) impairment of activities of daily living for spastic patients (Bottros & Christo, 2014).

▌ Diskography

Introduction

The intervertebral disks are innervated by the sinuvertebral nerve. This nerve has nociceptive and sympathetic innervation. Irritation and disruption of this nerve can cause pain. As such, the intervertebral disk can be a source of back pain. Internal disk disruption (IDD) is thought to be the most common cause of diskogenic pain. IDD results from disk degradation and development of radial fissures from the nucleus pulposus into the annulus fibrosus (Simon, McAuliffe, Shamim, Vuong, & Tahaei, 2014).

> ▶ **KEY POINT**
>
> A diskography is an interventional diagnostic procedure designed to assess integrity of the intervertebral disk.

This process entails puncture, stimulation, and assessment of the intervertebral disk. This procedure is the next step in the diagnostic algorithm if noninvasive diagnostic testing has not confirmed an etiology for a patient's presenting pain complaint (Manchikanti et al., 2003).

Clinical features

This pain may be described as deep/dull, associated with paraspinal muscle tightness, and worsens with Valsalva-type maneuvers (Simon et al., 2014).

Physical examination findings

On physical examination, pertinent findings include limited lumbar range of motion, kinesiophobia (fear of movement), and positive neural tension tests reproducing lower extremity or buttock pain (Simon et al., 2014).

> ▶ **KEY POINT**
>
> Intrinsic disk pain, also known as diskogenic pain, may present as predominant axial back or neck pain. There may be radicular or neuropathic pain that can radiate to the buttocks or lower extremity.

Interventional procedure type

Diskography is an outpatient interventional diagnostic procedure.

Brief description of procedure

The patient is placed prone for the procedure. Under fluoroscopic guidance, a radiopaque contrast is injected into the nucleus pulposus of the disk (Figure 9-8).

> ▶ **KEY POINT**
>
> The following information is collected: (1) identifying changes in morphology, (2) patient's concordant pain response, and (3) changes in pressure of the intervertebral disk as the contrast is injected.

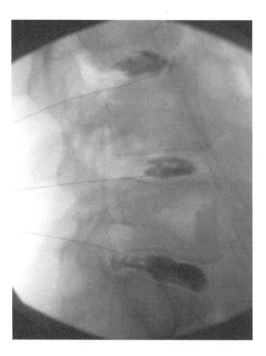

Figure 9–8. Diskography of L3-L4, L4-L5, and L5-S1.

The pressures are recorded via manometry. After the fluoroscopic diskogram procedure is completed, the patient has a spinal CT scan. This scan further elucidates the morphology of the tested intervertebral disks.

Contraindications

Contraindications to the procedure include: a patient unwilling to undergo the procedure, active infections, and bleeding disorders.

Risk/potential adverse effects

Complications for the procedure include infection (diskitis), neural trauma, intravascular penetration, and spinal cord trauma (Manchikanti et al., 2003).

Imaging modalities used to perform procedure

 KEY POINT

This interventional procedure is performed under fluoroscopic guidance. The postcontrast evaluation of the intervertebral disk is done under CT scan.

Type of medications used

Local anesthetic such as lidocaine may be used for superficial anesthesia. A radiopaque contrast, such as iohexol, is typically injected into the disk to obtain the information noted earlier. Frequently, an antibiotic (cephalosporin class) is injected as well to reduce the risk of postprocedural infection.

Sedations used

Typically, sedation is not used during this procedure as it may confound the diagnostic results.

Length of time for the procedure

Procedure may last between 30 minutes and 1 hour. The variance of time depends on the number of disks evaluated.

Expected postprocedural care

After the procedure, the patient is to avoid overly strenuous activity. The patient may have a few days of postprocedural soreness. After the procedure, it is important to monitor for signs of infection such as fevers or chills.

Frequency of having this procedure

The goal of the test is to determine if the intervertebral disk is the main etiology of a patient's pain compliant. During the course of the clinical workup, this procedure is typically performed once.

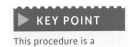

KEY POINT

This procedure is a diagnostic test.

Ways of documentation of efficacy

Documentation of treatment outcome can be done via (1) numeric rating scale, (2) modified Dallas Discogram Criteria, (3) American Medical Association (AMA) functional impairment guidelines, and (4) Oswestry Disability Index.

▌Neuropathic Pain Interventions

Neuropathic pain is pain resulting from damage to the peripheral nerves or to the central nervous system itself. More than 1.5 billion people worldwide suffer from chronic pain; approximately 3% to 4.5% of the global population suffers from neuropathic pain, with incidence rate increasing with age. Various interventional procedures are available for the treatment of this category of pain.

▌Neuropathic Pain: Peripheral Interventions

▌Peripheral Nerve Blocks

Introduction

Peripheral nerve blocks are utilized in acute situations, in surgical care, and to assist the management of persistent and chronic pain. The goal of these injections is to extinguish to nociceptive originating from a site of injury and to extinguish maladaptive neuropathic input from the nerves themselves (Garmon & O'Rourke, 2018).

Common targets of the upper quarter in chronic pain management include: median nerve, ulnar nerve, radial

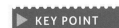

KEY POINT

Common nerve targets include cutaneous sensory nerves and motor nerves of both the upper and lower quarters of the body.

nerve, suprascapular nerve, and the intercostal nerves. Common targets of the lower quarter in chronic pain management include: lateral femoral cutaneous nerve, saphenous nerve, recurrent genicular nerve, ilioinguinal/iliohypogastric nerve, tibial nerve, and fibular nerve. Common facial and cranial nerve blocks are discussed in the head and neck section. Peripheral nerve blocks are commonly used in order to avoid systemic side effects of other medications and to decrease overall opioid use. Peripheral nerve blocks are a great alternative for anesthesia in an ambulatory setting especially as minimally invasive surgery technique continues to advance (Joshi, Gandhi, Shah, Gadsden, & Corman, 2016; Lin, Choi, & Hadzic, 2013).

Clinical features

The patient will typically describe paresthesia, hyperesthesia, allodynia, and anesthesia within the distribution of a peripheral nerve. Specifically, they will complain of a paroxysmal burning, tingling, numbness, and radiating pain. The patient may complain that specific compressive movements can increase the pain and that the pain is worse at night.

Physical examination findings

In general, the goal of the physical examination is to determine the specific involved peripheral nerve. This is done by determining topographically the dermatomal distribution of the complaint and testing for motor inhibition of the myotomes innervated by involved peripheral nerves. Two important physical examination tests to determine the dermatomal distribution are the (1) pinch and roll test for allodynia and (2) pinprick test for hyperesthesia. Special tests like Tinel's test can determine if there is any compressive influence on the nerve. Patient's history and physical examination findings will specify the nerve involved and the nerve's unique properties.

Interventional procedure type

Peripheral nerve blocks are an outpatient procedure. They are either (1) a single perineural injection or (2) a continuous infusion conducted via a perineural catheter.

Brief description of procedures/image modalities used

Procedure will vary depending on indication and target nerve. Different techniques may be employed for nerve guidance such as ultrasound, which may be used to identify superficial and deep nerves. Nerve stimulation may also be used to guide catheter or needle placement. Recent studies show ultrasound guidance is more cost-effective than nerve stimulation for continuous nerve block (Chang & White, 2017; Ehlers, Jensen, & Bendtsen, 2012).

Contraindications

Contraindications for this procedure are: (1) active local or systemic infection, (2) known neural defect at the target nerve, and (3) coagulopathy or anticoagulation use, especially if the nerve target is located within a fixed immobile site (Joshi et al., 2016).

Risk/potential adverse effects

Potential complications for this intervention include bleeding, bruising, systemic anesthetic toxicity, infection, direct nerve injury, and allergic reaction (Chang & White, 2017). The specific complications will depend where the injection is being performed.

Type of medications used

A combination of local anesthetic and steroid is used for peripheral nerve blockade. The local anesthetics are chosen depending on desired effect, intended duration of action, degree of motor blockade, and nerve target. Short-duration anesthetics include lidocaine and mepivacaine, whereas longer acting anesthetics include bupivacaine and ropivacaine. Corticosteroids are utilized for their anti-inflammatory effects (Wahal, Kumar, & Pyati, 2018).

Sedations used

Sedation is not used for this procedure.

Length of time for the procedure

Fifteen to 30 minutes.

Expected postprocedural care

The time for pain resolution for the peripheral nerve block will vary depending on steroid/anesthetic used and target nerve. Postprocedural numbness may last anywhere from 2 to 8 hours. Postprocedure patients should avoid high-intensity activity until they recover full motor and sensory function. Regular wound care should be applied to site (Joshi et al., 2016).

Frequency of having this procedure

Timing will vary depending on the indication for procedure, medication being used, target nerve, and practitioner preference.

Ways of documentation of efficacy

Documentation of treatment outcome can be done via (1) numeric rating scale, (2) visual analog scale, (3) functional measures, and (4) opioid consumption.

▌Peripheral Nerve Stimulation

Diagnosis/introduction

Similar to SCS, peripheral nerve stimulation (PNS) is a treatment modality for patients with intractable, chronic pain refractory to medical management. PNS involves the placement of a stimulating electrode over a peripheral nerve or plexus. There is a trial of the device followed by permanent placement.

Placement of the device upon the brachial plexus or the lumbar plexus can be done for a more general coverage of the upper and lower extremities (Goroszeniuk & Pang, 2014).

> ▶ **KEY POINT**
>
> Common nerves that undergo this procedure are occipital, supraorbital, infraorbital, radial, ulnar, median, tibial, peroneal, ilioinguinal, genitofemoral, and sciatic nerves (Chakravarthy, Nava, Christo, & Williams, 2016; Petersen & Slavin, 2014).

Clinical features

The patient will typically describe paresthesia, hyperesthesia, allodynia, and anesthesia within the distribution of a peripheral nerve. Specifically, they will complain of a paroxysmal burning, tingling, numbness, and radiating pain. There are several indications for PNS. These include neuropathic pain, chronic regional pain syndrome, facial pain, and cephalgia (specifically migraine, cluster headaches, and occipital headaches). Some recent indications for PNS include fibromyalgia and phantom limb pain (Chakravarthy et al., 2016; Petersen & Slavin, 2014).

Physical examination findings

As noted earlier for peripheral nerve blocks, the goal of physical examination is to determine the specific involved peripheral nerve. This is done by determining topographically the dermatomal distribution of the complaint and testing for motor inhibition of the myotomes innervated by involved peripheral nerves. Overall, the physical examination findings depend on the involved peripheral nerve.

Interventional procedure type

PNS trial is an outpatient interventional pain procedure. PNS implantation is a surgical procedure.

Brief description of the procedure

- ▶ PNS trial: The PNS trial involves placement of the electrode leads along the target nerve. The stimulation trial lasts for a defined time period ranging from 2 to 14 days.
- ▶ PNS placement: Under fluoroscopy/ultrasound, the patient is appropriately positioned and the skin is cleaned and draped. Local anesthetic is injected superficially. A Tuohy needle is advanced in the subcutaneous space overlying the nerve. The electrode lead is threaded in and the position is confirmed by imaging. At this point, the stimulation can be tested and the patient may report the area of coverage. The electrode is then anchored to the fascia with sutures. The generator device is then implanted subcutaneously (Petersen & Slavin, 2014).

Contraindications

Contraindications for this procedure include: active infection, immunocompromised patients, anticoagulation, bleeding disorders, cognitive impairment, untreated psychiatric disease, and malingering (Petersen & Slavin, 2014).

Risk/potential adverse effects

Complications from this procedure may include infection, lead erosion, migration of the lead, or mechanical issues with the device. The most common complication is lead migration (Deer et al., 2014). Neural injury is a rare but serious complication (Petersen & Slavin, 2014).

Imaging modalities used to perform procedure

PNS trial and placement is performed under fluoroscopic guidance (Chan, Brown, Park, & Winfree, 2010).

Type of medications used

Local anesthesia is typically administered for this procedure.

Sedations used

Conscious sedation may be used during stimulation trial in certain cases. Implantation of the permanent stimulator device is typically done under general anesthesia (Petersen & Slavin, 2014).

Length of time for the procedure

Generally, the procedure takes 30 minutes to 1 hour to perform. The time duration varies depending on the involved nerve or plexus.

Expected postprocedural care

Postprocedurally, the patients should refrain from strenuous activity. An antibiotic may be administered prophylactically (Petersen & Slavin, 2014). The electrode cables that are laid externally should be kept clean and dry.

Frequency of having this procedure

After a PNS trial and permanent device placement, further procedures are typically not performed unless a revision is needed.

Ways of documentation of efficacy

Documentation of treatment outcome can be done via (1) numeric rating scale, (2) visual analog pain scale, and (3) Migraine Disability Assessment score (Goroszeniuk & Pang, 2014).

▌Peripheral Nerve Hydrodissection

Introduction

Hydrodissection employs the technique of using fluid at high pressure to separate or "dissect out" a particular tissue layer with the goal of pain relief by means of fascial decompression and creating new surgical planes (Lam, Reeves, & Cheng, 2017).

Common nerve entrapment sites include the median nerve at the wrist, radial nerve as it traverses through the supinator muscle, or ulnar nerve at the elbow. Multiple peripheral nerve and deep nerve structures may be accessed for this procedure such as brachial plexus and stellate ganglion (Cass, 2016).

> ▶ **KEY POINT**
>
> Initially being used during surgical procedures in order to preserve neuronal structures, this technique is now performed to treat different pain diagnoses such as chronic neuropathic pain and nerve entrapment, such as can be seen with scleroderma or nerve compression.

> ▶ **KEY POINT**
>
> Selecting the correct interventional pain procedure depends on the patient's diagnosis, treatment indications, and potential contraindications.

Clinical features

Neuropathic pain patients will describe their pain as burning type that may be accompanied by numbness and tingling, which may or may not follow a particular nerve distribution (Rowlingson, 2005). Symptoms of nerve entrapment include pain and paresthesia along a particular nerve distribution. Common nerve entrapment sites include: median nerve entrapment at the wrist that involves the first three digits and lateral aspect of the palm, ulnar nerve entrapment at the elbow involving the fourth and fifth digits along with medial aspect of palm, ulnar nerve entrapment at the supinator or radial groove of the humerus that will affect the dorsum or hand and posterior forearm (Buchanan & Dulebohn, 2018; Kowalska & Sudoł-Szopińska, 2012).

Physical examination findings

Examination for neuropathic pain is often nonspecific and noncontributory but nerve entrapment will present with particular findings on examination. Median nerve entrapment will present with weak grip strength and thumb abduction along with wasting of thenar eminence. Tinel's sign (tapping on volar aspect of wrist reproduces symptoms) and Phalen's maneuver (flexion of wrist causing dysesthesias) may be positive. Nocturnal paresthesia is reported as being the most sensitive clinical sign (Meyer et al., 2018). Ulnar nerve entrapment will present with weak fifth finger abduction and wasting of hypothenar musculature. Tinel's sign at the elbow may also be positive. Although less commonly encountered clinically, radial nerve entrapment will have weak triceps, wrist and/or finger extension depending on the level of entrapment (Buchanan & Dulebohn, 2018).

Interventional Procedure Type

This is an outpatient procedure.

Brief description of procedure for this diagnosis

Procedure is done under ultrasound guidance, which may be performed in the out-of-plane technique (needle is parallel to the ultrasound probe) or the in-plane technique (needle is perpendicular to the probe). After prepping the skin in an aseptic manner, the particular nerve will be localized. Hypoechoic landmarks on ultrasound (cartilage appears hypoechoic, whereas blood vessels appear black or anechoic) are traced until the area of pathology is identified. Using known hypoechoic landmarks on ultrasound (cartilage appears hypoechoic, whereas blood vessels appear black or anechoic) and will be traced until area of suspected pathology. Short bursts of high-pressure fluid are then used to advance needle through the area of suspected entrapment, effectively freeing the nerve from the surrounding fascia and subcutaneous tissue (Cass, 2016). Once this is achieved, the needle is removed and the procedure is concluded.

Contraindications

Include allergy to medication, bleeding diathesis, therapeutic anticoagulation, and overlying skin infection. Known anatomic abnormalities that would impede appropriate needle maneuvering may also be a contraindication.

Risk/potential adverse effects

As with any injection, common side effects include bruising, bleeding, and infections at the injection site. Other specific side effects for this procedure include neural injury or unintentional neural trespass (Cass, 2016).

Imaging modalities used to perform procedure

Procedure is performed under ultrasound guidance. Ultrasound provides visualization of the neurovascular structures. Ultrasound is a dynamic tool, which provides real-time needle placement in order to undergo successful release of the entrapped nerve (Lam, Reeves, & Cheng, 2017).

Type of medications used

Procedure is most commonly done using 5% dextrose although some practitioners commonly use local anesthetic such as lidocaine in order to anesthetize the needle tract (Lam, Reeves, & Cheng, 2017).

Sedations used

Sedation is not typically done with this procedure.

Length of time for the procedure

Fifteen to 30 minutes.

Expected postprocedural care

The patient is to avoid strenuous activity 24 to 48 hours after injection.

Frequency of having this procedure

There is no consensus on how many procedures may be done in a set period of time. Repeated nerve hydrodissections are discouraged because of the risk of nerve injury.

Ways of documentation of efficacy

Documentation of treatment outcome can be done via (1) visual analog scale and (2) numeric pain rating scale (Lam, Reeves, & Cheng, 2017).

Neuropathic Pain: Central Interventions

Deep Brain Stimulation

Introduction

Deep brain stimulation (DBS) is an interventional procedure commonly used in movement disorders, which can also be used for chronic pain retractable to medical management. It works by delivering an electrical current through implanted electrodes in the intracranial space at subcortical targets thought to be involved in the specific pain syndrome. These targets include the periaqueductal/periventricular gray, sensory thalamic nuclei (ventral posteromedial nucleus, ventral posterolateral nucleus), anterior cingulate cortex, internal capsule, globus pallidus, and other structures involved in the physiology of pain (Boccard, Pereira, & Aziz, 2015; Falowski, 2015).

KEY POINT

There are multiple indications for DBS. These include neuropathic pain, facial pain, FBSS, phantom limb pain, poststroke pain, brachial plexus avulsion, trigeminal nerve pain, cephalalgias, and headache disorders (Boccard, Pereira, & Aziz, 2015; Falowski, 2015).

Diagnosis key patient history/symptoms presentation

As previously mentioned, presentation may differ depending on the pain disorder.

Diagnosis key physical examination findings

Vary depending on the pain disorder.

Interventional procedure type

This is a surgical procedure.

Brief description of procedure for this diagnosis

The skin is cleaned and draped. A unilateral burr hole is prepared to accommodate the target through a transfrontal extraventricular trajectory on or near the coronal suture. Intraoperative electrode stimulation is done on the target to elicit sensation in the desired distribution. The lead is then implanted and secured. After a successful postoperative trial, the patient is then brought back for internalization and placement of an implantable pulse generator that is connected to the lead cable subcutaneously (Ben-Haim, Mirzadeh, & Rosenberg, 2018).

Contraindications

Contraindications for DBS include: biologic age over 75 years, severe or malignant comorbidity with reduced life expectancy, chronic immunosuppression, distinct brain atrophy, and severe psychological disorder (Groiss, Wojtecki, Südmeyer, & Schnitzler, 2009).

Risk/potential adverse effects

There are a wide range of complications from DBS device placement. The more serious complications include intracranial hemorrhage and permanent neurologic deficits. Other complications include infection, transient headaches, diplopia, nausea, vertical gaze palsies, blurred vision, and nystagmus (Falowski, 2015).

Imaging modalities used to perform procedure

CT and MRI of the head are typically done before and after the surgical procedure (Ben-Haim, Mirzadeh, & Rosenberg, 2018).

Type of medications used

Superficial local anesthetic is given. Intravenous anesthetic is given intraoperatively.

Sedations used

Electrode placement requires the patient to be awake. However, impulse generator implantation is done under general anesthesia.

Length of time for the procedure

Depends on the technique used, but may last between 3 and 6 hours.

Expected postprocedural care

Patients are typically hospitalized for close monitoring.

Frequency of having this procedure for this diagnosis

Typically, this procedure is performed once. The patient, however, may need surgical revisions.

Ways of documentation of efficacy

Documentation of treatment outcome can be done via (1) visual analog scale, (2) health-related quality of life, (3) McGill pain questionnaire (MPQ), and (4) pain disability index.

Neuropathic Pain: Sympathetic Interventions

Sympathetic Blocks

Introduction

The autonomic nervous system comprises the parasympathetic and sympathetic systems that work together to maintain homeostasis. Dysfunction of the sympathetic nervous system, primarily responsible for the "fight or flight" response, will result in uncontrolled sympathetic flow leading to significant pain and dysfunction. The sympathetic chain is located lateral to the vertebral body and runs through the entirety of the spine and may be blocked at multiple levels. Commonly performed sympathetic blocks include stellate ganglion block (Figure 9-9), celiac plexus block, lumbar sympathetic block (Figure 9-10), and hypogastric plexus block.

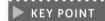
▶ **KEY POINT**

Indications for sympathetic block are chronic lower limb pain, phantom limb pain, CRPSs, chronic pelvic and perineal pain, and zoster infection.

Figure 9-9. Stellate ganglion block.

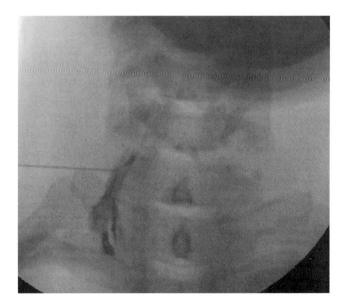

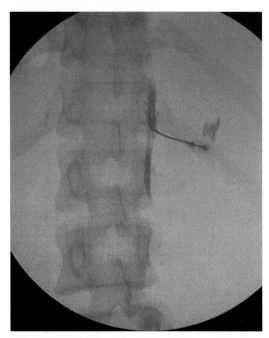

Figure 9–10. Lumbar sympathetic block.

Although less common, there have been case reports for its use in refractory painful diabetic neuropathy, lumbar hyperhidrosis, and erythromelalgia (Alexander & Dulebohn, 2018).

Clinical features

Specific findings will depend on the underlying etiology but common descriptions of pain in sympathetic dysfunction include paresthesia and dysesthesias, which are commonly accompanied by swelling, temperature changes, muscles spasms, hyperhidrosis, and erythema of the affected extremity. This can be noted on physical examination by comparing the affected to the unaffected side (Bruehl, 2015).

Interventional procedure type

The paravertebral sympathetic ganglion injection is an outpatient procedure.

Brief description of procedure for this diagnosis

Patient is positioned under fluoroscopic machine and skin prepped in an aseptic manner. Under fluoroscopy guidance, the desired level is located and endplates are aligned. On oblique view, transverse processes are aligned with anterior aspect of vertebral body. Needle is directed toward anterior aspect of vertebral body. Placement is confirmed with contrast and anterior posterior view of the fluoroscopy machine (Waldam, 2006).

Contraindications

Contraindications for this procedure are systemic anticoagulation, allergies to medications used, uncontrolled.

Risk/potential adverse effects

Common side effects include bruising, bleeding, swelling, pain at injection site, and orthostatic hypotension. Other complications include infection, intravascular spread of medication, and allergic reaction to medication. Given proximity of sympathetic chain to the vascular structures, there is an increased risk of vascular injury and significant hemorrhage (Waldam, 2006).

Imaging modalities used to perform procedure

Procedure is performed under fluoroscopy, ultrasound, or CT guidance (Baig, Moon, & Shankar, 2017).

Type of medications used

Neurolytic procedures are performed with alcohol or phenol, and RFA may also be used. Botulinum toxin has also been used in the treatment of CRPS (Carroll, Clark, & Mackey, 2009).

Sedations used

Sedation is not used for this procedure.

Length of time for the procedure

Fifteen to 30 minutes.

Expected postprocedural care

Postprocedural care includes: regular wound care and avoidance of water submersion for first 24 to 48 hours. Careful monitoring is done given possible side effects from sympathetic blockade.

Frequency of having this procedure

There is no consensus on optimal timing between procedures, but the timing will depend on patient's response to procedure and the physician's preference.

Ways of documentation of efficacy

Documentation of treatment outcome can be done via (1) visual analog scale, (2) functional status, and (3) quality of life scale.

Orthopedic Pain Interventions

Orthopedic pain involves pain originating from the articular structures of the extremities. These structures can be large joints, like the hip and shoulder, or smaller joints like the subacromial bursa or the digits of the hand. Reducing the nociceptive pain from joints can help with improved patient functionality and in turn increased participation in physical therapy and other therapeutic environments.

Orthopedic Pain: Intraarticular Joint Interventions

Diagnosis/introduction

Most, if not all, peripheral and axial joints are accessible for injection but most commonly intraarticular joint injections include wrist, elbow, shoulder, hip, and knee. Osteoarthritis also known as degenerative joint disease is typically attributed to "wear and tear" of a joint over time, involving loss of articular cartilage. Rheumatoid arthritis is part of a chronic generalized autoimmune process that involves a wide variety of symptoms, with joint involvement resulting from synovial inflammation and subsequent joint degradation (Cheng, Souzdalnitski, Vrooman, & Cheng, 2012; Paterson et al., 2018).

> ▶ **KEY POINT**
>
> Precise determination of the source of pain, via physical examination and diagnostic evaluation, is key in identifying the correct anatomic treatment target and planning proper interventional treatment.

> ▶ **KEY POINT**
>
> Intraarticular joint injections have been a mainstay of treatment for osteoarthritis, rheumatoid arthritis, and other inflammatory arthropathies for many years.

Diagnosis of key patient history

Hallmark symptom for osteoarthritis is pain with ambulation or movement, which is usually alleviated by rest; other commonly encountered symptoms include stiffness late in the day, asymmetric joint involvement described as "hard and bony," with an overall lack of systemic symptoms. Classical findings on imaging for osteoarthritis include: joint space narrowing, osteophyte formation, subchondral sclerosis, and subchondral cysts (Swagerty & Hellinger, 2001). On the other hand, rheumatoid arthritis will present with significant morning stiffness, symmetric joint involvement usually described as "swollen and warm." Patients with rheumatoid arthritis may also report extraarticular involvement such as fever, fatigue, or other autoimmune conditions (Liow, Wang, & Loh, 2017).

Key physical examination findings

Patients with osteoarthritis will present with asymmetric joint involvement with crepitus, bony tenderness, and enlargement, which may be seen on physical examination. Involvement of distal interphalangeal joints is classic for osteoarthritis, which are known as Heberden's nodes (Liow, Wang, & Loh, 2017). Physical presentation for rheumatoid arthritis may be varied depending on extent of disease at presentation but will likely have polyarticular involvement. Joints are involved symmetrically and will preferentially affect metacarpophalangeal joint and proximal interphalangeal joint, which are known as Bouchard nodes (Turesson, O'Fallon, Crowson, Gabriel, & Matteson, 2003).

Interventional procedure type

Intraarticular injections are an outpatient procedure.

Brief description of procedure for this diagnosis

Most commonly injected joints include knee, shoulder (Figure 9-11), and hip (Figure 9-12). There are various techniques available to access peripheral joints, and the overall approach will depend on practitioner's preference, availability of imaging options (such as ultrasound or fluoroscopy), patient comfort, and presence of a joint effusion. Local anesthetic such as lidocaine may be used to anesthetize the needle tract in order to improve patient comfort during the procedure. Practitioner will then proceed to perform injection, carefully guiding the needle into the joint space in order to deliver the medication. This may or may not be done with or without image guidance (Maricar, Parkes, Callaghan, Felson, & O'Neill, 2013).

Contraindications

Contraindications include allergy to medication being injected or particular antiseptic skin preparation being used, bleeding diathesis, therapeutic anticoagulation, uncontrolled diabetes, and local skin infection.

Risk/potential adverse effects

Adverse effects include worsening pain and swelling at the injection site, bruising, bleeding, and overlying skin infection. Other more serious side effects including septic arthritis, necrotizing fasciitis, intravascular spread of medication, and even cases of air embolism have been reported in the literature (Cheng & Abdi, 2007).

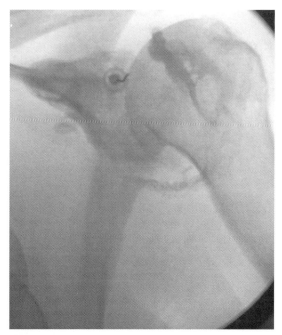

Figure 9–11. Intraarticular joint injection of the shoulder.

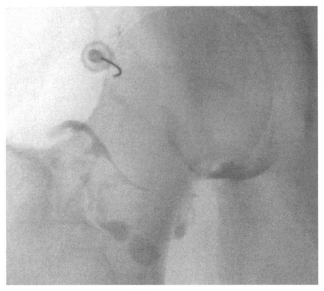

Figure 9-12. Intraarticular joint injection of the hip.

Imaging modalities used to perform procedure

This greatly improves the diagnostic accuracy of the procedure as well as avoiding serious adverse effects such as nerve and/or vascular injury. Review of the current literature available shows that the use of some form of image guidance compared to landmark-based guidance will result in increased accuracy of the intraarticular injections across multiple joints (Daniels, Cole, Jacobs, & Phillips, 2018).

Type of medications used

There are many different medications that may be injected into any peripheral joint. Most commonly, a mixture of local anesthetic (such as lidocaine or bupivacaine) and corticosteroid (such as triamcinolone, methylprednisolone, or dexamethasone) is used both for their long-term and short-term analgesic effects (Jüni et al., 2015). Intraarticular hyaluronic acid, also known as viscosupplementation, is used with the intent of restoring viscoelastic properties of synovial fluids. Other more novel alternatives include platelet-rich plasma, prolotherapy, and even adipose-derived pluripotent cells (Ayhan, Kesmezacar, & Akgun, 2014).

Sedations used

Sedation is not commonly used for these procedures.

Length of time for the procedure

Fifteen to 30 minutes.

Expected postprocedural care

Regular wound care should be applied; avoid strenuous activity and submerging injection site in water during the first 24 to 48 hours. Some particular medications such as adipose transfer procedure may have specific postprocedure care protocol.

Frequency of having this procedure

Given concerns for systemic side effects of glucocorticoids, practitioners will limit intraarticular steroid injections to less than four injections per year and not more frequent than every 6 weeks.

Ways of documentation of efficacy

Documentation of treatment outcome can be done via (1) visual analog scale, (2) functional impairment score, (3) Lequesne indices, and (4) Western Ontario and McMaster Universities Osteoarthritis (WOMAC) index (Dawson et al., 2005).

▌ Orthopedic Pain: Bursa Injections

Diagnosis/Introduction

Bursa injections are often performed in the setting of localized bursitis with abnormality of the adjacent tendon (Adler & Sofka, 2003).

> ▶ **KEY POINT**
>
> The most commonly performed bursa injections are the subacromial and greater trochanteric bursa injections.

Diagnosis of key patient history/symptoms presentation

- ▷ Subacromial bursitis: Subacromial bursitis typically develops in throwing athletes and presents as anterior shoulder pain and shoulder range of motion restriction. A painful arc syndrome, similar to impingement symptoms, may occur (Chen et al., 2006). Injections are usually done if conservative treatment is unsuccessful.
- ▷ Greater trochanteric bursitis: Greater trochanteric bursitis is one of the conditions within greater trochanteric pain syndrome. Presentation includes lateral hip pain that is worse with pressure on that side of the body. Pain occurs with walking or while standing on affected leg (Mallow & Nazarian, 2014). Greater trochanteric bursa injections are performed if conservative measures are ineffective and if bursitis is thought to be the etiology of the pain (Payne, 2016).

Physical examination findings

- ▷ Subacromial bursitis: Reproduction of index pain with palpation over the subacromial bursa (Chen et al., 2006) and shoulder abduction.

▶ Greater trochanteric bursitis: Reproduction of index pain with direct palpation on the greater trochanter and with resisted abduction with external rotation (Mallow & Nazarian, 2014).

Interventional procedure type
These intrabursal injection procedures are done in an outpatient setting.

Brief description of procedure for this diagnosis
▶ Subacromial bursa injection:
  ● Anterior approach: Under ultrasound guidance, the probe is positioned on the axial plane of the front of the shoulder and the needle is inserted into the lateromedial direction (Molini, Mariacher, & Bianchi, 2012).
  ● Superior approach: Under ultrasound guidance, the probe is positioned in the supraspinatus fossa, parallel to the axis of the supraspinatus muscle with the lateral edge over the acromion (Molini, Mariacher, & Bianchi, 2012).
  ● Posterior approach: After the posterolateral corner of the acromion is identified, the skin is entered one finger-breadth inferior, with the needle slightly medial and cephalad (Monseau & Nizran, 2013).
  ● Lateral approach: After the lateral border of the acromion is identified, the skin is injected one finger-breadth inferior to the midway point of the lateral border of the acromion, with the needle perpendicular to the border to the acromion. If ultrasound guidance is done, the probe is positioned parallel to the long axis of the supraspinatus. The lateral approach is more commonly performed under ultrasound guidance (Molini, Mariacher, & Bianchi, 2012).
▶ Greater trochanteric bursa (Figure 9-13):
  ● With patient in the appropriate position, the skin is cleansed and draped. Local anesthetic is injected. Under imaging or anatomic landmark guidance, the needle is entered perpendicular to the table until bone is reached. The medication is then administered (Monseau & Nizran, 2013).

Contraindications
Absolute contraindications include hypersensitivity, active infection, uncontrolled bleeding disorder, prosthetic/unstable joint, and intraarticular fracture (Monseau & Nizran, 2013).

Risk/potential adverse effects
As with many injections, complications include infections, septic arthritis, bleeding, and local bruises (Molini, Mariacher, & Bianchi, 2012).

Imaging modalities used to perform procedure
The procedure is typically performed under ultrasound or fluoroscopic guidance (Payne, 2016).

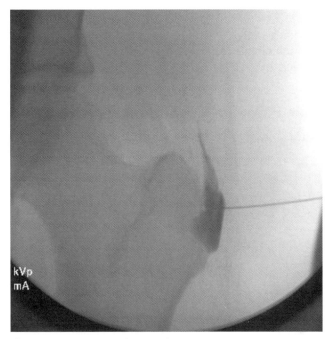

Figure 9–13. Greater trochanteric bursa.

Type of medications used

Typically, a mixture of local anesthetic (such as lidocaine) and steroids is used. Commonly used steroids include methylprednisolone, triamcinolone, betamethasone, and dexamethasone (Monseau & Nizran, 2013).

Sedations used

Sedation is typically not done, although this may depend on the provider and patient.

Length of time for the procedure

Between 30 minutes and 1 hour, although this may vary depending on the patient and provider.

Expected postprocedural care

▶ Supraspinatus bursa injection: Patients are advised to avoid shoulder load for 2 to 3 days.
▶ Greater trochanter injection: Relative rest, avoid strenuous activity, monitor for signs of infection.

Frequency of having this procedure for this diagnosis

These procedures may be repeated if they provide pain relief. However, prolonged steroid use may affect the surrounding tendons.

Ways of documentation of efficacy

Documentation of treatment outcome can be done via (1) visual analog pain scale, (2) Oswestry Disability Index, (3) short form 36 scores, and (4) reduction in analgesic use.

Orthopedic Pain: Soft Tissue Interventions

Piriformis Injection

Introduction

The piriformis muscle is the only muscle that courses transversely through the greater sciatic notch (Jankovic, Peng, & Zundert, 2013).

It is a common cause of buttock and leg pain.

> **▶ KEY POINT**
>
> Piriformis syndrome is defined as a nondiskogenic cause of sciatica because of impingement of the sciatic nerve through or around the piriformis muscle (Cass, 2015).

Clinical features

Presentation can be insidious or due to injury. Patients report buttock pain with or without lower extremity pain. There may be associated back, groin, perineum, or hip pain (Jankovic, Peng, & Zundert, 2013).

Physical examination findings

On physical examination, there is tenderness upon palpation of the piriformis muscle.

> **▶ KEY POINT**
>
> There is pain on passive forced internal rotation and adduction of the hip in supine position (Freiberg's maneuver). Lastly, there may be pain on adduction, flexion, and internal rotation of the lower extremity (Jankovic, Peng, & Zundert, 2013; Michel et al., 2013).

Interventional procedure type

This procedure is an outpatient intramuscular injection.

Brief description of procedure

Piriformis injections are performed when patients fail conservative modalities such as physical therapy, lifestyle modification, or pharmacologic agents. For ultrasound-guided procedures, the gluteal region on the affected side is scanned with a long linear ultrasound transducer. Bony acoustic landmarks are used to localize the course of the piriformis muscle. Once the skin is cleaned and marked, the needle is inserted from medial to lateral, parallel to the long axis of the piriformis, using an in-plane technique on ultrasound (Smith, Hurdle, Locketz, & Wisniewski, 2006). The procedure can also be performed under fluoroscopic guidance.

Contraindications

Contraindications for this procedure include active infection, allergic reaction, and anticoagulation use or bleeding disorders (Simons, Travell, & Travell, 1999).

Risk/potential adverse effects

The potential adverse effects are sciatic nerve injury, infection, and bleeding.

Imaging modalities used to perform procedure

Imaging modalities for this injection include ultrasound, fluoroscopy (Figure 9-14), CT, and MRI. The accuracy of needle placement with ultrasound was 95% on a cadaveric study (Finoff, Hurdle, & Smith, 2008). In addition, electromyography localization may be used with a monopolar needle.

Type of medications used

Long-acting corticosteroids such as methylprednisolone or triamcinolone are regularly used (Johansson, 1990). Local anesthetics such as lidocaine or bupivacaine may be injected in conjunction during this procedure. More recently, the use of botulinum toxin is gaining popularity (Kirschner, Foye, & Cole, 2009).

Sedations used

Sedation is not used for this procedure.

Length of time for the procedure

Fifteen to 30 minutes.

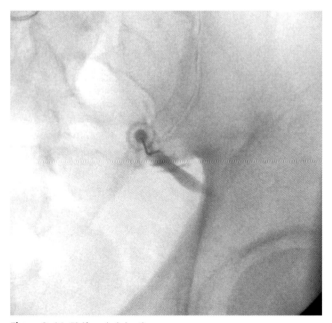

Figure 9–14. Piriformis injection.

Expected postprocedural care

Postprocedurally, patients should avoid high-intensity activity and avoid submersion of injection site. There may be some soreness and temporary flare of symptoms can be expected (Smith, Hurdle, Locketz, & Wisniewski, 2006).

Frequency of having this procedure

The number of times the procedure is done depends on the patient's symptom severity, the reactions to previous injection, and the provider's preference. The range may be once every 3 to 4 months.

Ways of documentation of efficacy

Documentation of treatment outcome can be done via (1) visual analog scale and (2) numeric rating scale.

Myofascial Trigger Point Injection

Introduction

Myofascial trigger points (MTPs) are defined as discrete, palpable nodules in a taut band of skeletal muscle that cause referred pain upon compression (Shah et al., 2015). Trigger point injections (TPIs) are performed when conservative treatments such as massage therapy or physical therapy are unsuccessful.

Clinical features

Myofascial pain can be caused by postural changes and associated with restrictive range of motion. They can occur spontaneously or as a result of injury. Patients usually have focal pain with discrete referral patterns (Borg-Stein & Iaccarino, 2014). This condition may be associated with muscle spasm, stiffness, decreased range of motion, and autonomic dysfunction (Espejo-Antinez et al., 2017).

> ▶ **KEY POINT**
>
> The mechanism of action is that the needle mechanically disrupts and stops the dysfunctional activity of the motor end plate of the skeletal muscle motor neuron (Borg-Stein & Iaccarino, 2014).

Physical examination findings

Palpation perpendicular to the muscle fibers is used to identify the MTP. It should produce significant pain, reproducing the patient's symptoms (Borg-Stein & Iaccarino, 2014).

Interventional procedure type

TPIs are an outpatient procedure.

> ▶ **KEY POINT**
>
> Some studies have shown improved success with a local twitch response (Chu, 1995).

Brief description of procedure

An MTP is identified by reproduction of the indexed pain or a local twitch response with palpation. After cleaning the surrounding skin, a small-gauge needle is inserted into the trigger point. The muscle and surrounding fascia are then probed with an up and down motion of the needle in a clockwise direction (Shah et al., 2015).

Contraindications

Contraindications to the procedure include active infection, allergic reaction, and anticoagulation usage or bleeding disorders (Simons, Travell, & Travell, 1999).

Risk/potential adverse effects

Although TPIs are generally considered safe, serious complications have been reported based on the location of the injection. These complications include pneumothorax, intrathecal injection, epidural abscess, and skeletal muscle toxicity (Cheng & Abdi, 2007).

Imaging modalities used to perform procedure

TPIs are usually done without any imaging modalities. Ultrasound may be considered in some cases (Shah et al., 2015).

Type of medications used

Local anesthetics such as lidocaine, procaine, or bupivacaine may be injected for this procedure. Steroids and botulinum toxin A have been shown to provide pain relief (Kietrys et al., 2013; Majlesi & Unalan, 2010). The evidence for the utilization of steroid or Botox in TPIs is limited (Borg-Stein & Iaccarino, 2014).

Sedations used

Sedation is not used for this procedure.

Length of time for the procedure

Fifteen to 30 minutes.

Expected postprocedural care

 KEY POINT

After the TPI, a patient may experience a localized soreness in the area of injection. This can last a few days and is self-resolving.

Frequency of having this procedure

TPIs are typically performed weekly over a series of several visits (Borg-Stein & Iaccarino, 2014). The total number of visits and treatment frequency is individually determined by the provider.

Ways of documentation of efficacy

Documentation of treatment outcome can be done via (1) visual analog scale, (2) AMA impairment guidelines, specifically cervical range of motion, and (3) analgesic intake (Espejo-Antunez et al., 2017).

▌Headache/Face Pain Interventions

Headache and facial pain are often debilitating conditions for patients. Trigeminal neuralgia and migraines are two such conditions. Fortunately, there are interventional procedures that can be used to treat these conditions.

▌Trigeminal Nerve Blocks

Introduction

The trigeminal nerve, named for its three divisions, is the fifth and largest cranial nerve. This nerve supplies sensory innervation to the face and motor function to the muscles of mastication (Zakrzewska & McMillan, 2011). Trigeminal neuralgia is a chronic neuropathic pain condition. Commonly, trigeminal neuralgia involves extraneural compression by surrounding vasculature, tumor, or arteriovenous malformations (Cruccu et al., 2016). Other indications for trigeminal nerve block include herpes zoster infection of the face, also known as zoster ophthalmicus.

Clinical features

Trigeminal neuralgia is a neuropathic pain condition. Patients may complain of paroxysmal paresthesia in the distribution of the trigeminal nerve along the face. Pain episodes last a few seconds to a couple of minutes and occur multiple times a day. Patient descriptors may include sharp, shooting pain and electric shocks. Specific distribution of symptoms will vary depending on which nerve divisions are affected (Maarbjerg, Di Stefano, Bendtsen, & Cruccu, 2017).

Physical examination findings

Patient will often avoid any stimulus that might trigger their pain; hence, they may appear guarded during physical examination. Careful sensory and motor examination should be performed. The physical examination may be normal given that episodes are usually paroxysmal in origin (Maarbjerg, Di Stefano, Bendtsen, & Cruccu, 2017).

Interventional procedure type

Trigeminal nerve blocks are an outpatient peripheral perineural injection or ganglion blockade.

Brief description of procedure for this diagnosis

The trigeminal nerve blocks are employed when more conservative approaches prove ineffective. The trigeminal nerve can be blocked at the level of the trigeminal ganglia or peripherally as the nerves exit the skill to innervate the skin (Cruccu et al., 2008). The particular branches of the trigeminal nerve are the ophthalmic, mandibular, and maxillary division. The nerve targets of the blocks depend on the patient's underlying diagnosis (Moskovitz & Sabatino, 2013).

Ophthalmic block

The superior orbital or the supratrochlear nerve may be targeted as they each exit around the ocular orbit. To target the supratrochlear nerve, specifically, the medication is injected at approximately 17 and 27 mm from the glabellar midline, respectively.

Maxillary block

The maxillary division is targeted using multiple approaches depending on practitioner comfort and experience. With the external approach, the needle is inserted below the zygomatic arch between the coronoid and condyle of the mandible and guided up till the pterygopalatine fossa is reached. Both the high-tuberosity approach and the great palatine canal approach are performed through the inside of the mouth in order to reach the pterygopalatine fossa.

Mandibular block

The main target location is the posterior branch of the mandibular nerve. This branch carries the sensory input. The patient is asked to open the mouth and the needle is inserted below the zygomatic arch at the midpoint of the arch of the mandible; at the level of the pterygoid plate, the needle is directed posteriorly toward the ear.

Trigeminal ganglion block

The needle is inserted medially to the ramus of the mandible and guided posteriorly toward the foramen ovale. The ultimate needle placement is then confirmed with imaging.

Contraindications

Contraindications to this procedure are an allergy to local anesthetic, an allergy to the injectate, active infection, and a known anatomic variation that prohibits the delivery of medication.

Risk/potential adverse effects

Adverse effects include facial paralysis, cephalgia, bruising, and infections. Unintentional neural damage or perforation may also occur. Hematomas may occur after external approach of the maxillary block. Epidural placement of medication may result in brainstem anesthesia and/or seizures. Diplopia and eye lid edema may be seen with ophthalmic blocks. Patients may experience troublesome dysesthesias or anesthesia dolorosa (Cruccu et al., 2008; Maarbjerg, Di Stefano, Bendtsen, & Cruccu, 2017).

Imaging modalities used to perform procedure

Peripheral procedures may be performed without image guidance based on anatomic landmarks. Commonly, trigeminal ganglion blockade is performed under fluoroscopic, ultrasound, or CT guidance.

Type of medications used

Therapeutic peripheral blocks use local anesthetic such as lidocaine or bupivacaine. Neurolytic procedures use alcohol, phenol, or glycerol. Ganglion blocks may use glycerol to induce neurolysis.

Sedations used

No sedation is needed for peripheral blockade but a ganglion blockade may require sedation.

Length of time for the procedure

The duration of the procedure is generally 15 to 30 minutes.

Expected postprocedural care

After the procedure, the patient should be monitored for any signs of infection or changes/deterioration in neurologic function.

Ways of documentation of efficacy

Documentation of treatment outcome can be done via (1) numeric rating scale, (2) visual analog scale, (3) brief pain index—facial scale, (5) Initiative on Methods, Measurement and Pain Assessment in Clinical Trials (IMMPACT), (6) MPQ, and (7) Barrow Neurological Institute pain intensity score (Kumar, Rastogi, Mahendra, Bansal, & Chandra, 2017).

Botox Injections

Introduction

Intramuscular administration of onabotulinum toxin A (Botox) recently was approved by the Food and Drug Administration (FDA) for use in the prevention of chronic migraine. It is also approved by the FDA to treat cervical dystonia and torticollis. The proposed mechanism of action involves the inhibition of calcitonin gene–related peptide and substance P release in synapse vesicles in the trigeminovascular system (Whitcup, Turkel, DeGryse, & Brin, 2014).

> ▶ **KEY POINT**
>
> Interventional pain treatment uses techniques such as nerve blocks and chemodenervation to directly address the source of a patient's pain.

Clinical features

Migraine headaches present with unilateral, throbbing, pulsating pain accompanied by nausea, vomiting, photophobia, and phonophobia. The headache may be preceded by an aura. Prodromal and postdromal symptoms may also be present, which include hyperactivity, hypoactivity, depression, cravings for particular foods, repetitive yawning, fatigue, and neck stiffness and/or pain. Migraines can become chronic if they present for 15 or more days a month for more than 3 months (Headache Classification Committee of the International Headache Society [IHS], 2013).

Physical examination findings

Migraines can present with reversible neurologic deficits such as hemiplegia, visual defects, dysarthria, and ataxia. Patients typically do not have any focal neurologic findings on examination if they are not actively having a migraine or aura (IHS, 2013).

Interventional procedure type

This procedure is an outpatient intramuscular injection.

Brief description of procedure

After proper positioning, the skin is cleaned and draped. A small-gauge needle is inserted at a 45° angle to the plane of the head and neck.

A total of 200 units of onabotulinum toxin A is divided among each muscle site (Szok, Csáti, Vécsei, & Tajti, 2015).

> ▶ **KEY POINT**
>
> There is a standardized technique where 31 sites located on the head and neck regions are injected. These sites include the bilateral corrugator, procerus, frontalis, temporalis, occipitalis, cervical paraspinal, and trapezius muscles.

Contraindications

Contraindications for this procedure include systemic infection or infection at injection site, hypersensitivity or allergy to onabotulinum toxin A, and history of neuromuscular junction disease such as myasthenia gravis.

Risk/potential adverse effects

Documented adverse effects from botulinum toxin injections include: increased neck pain, muscular weakness, musculoskeletal stiffness, ptosis, swallowing problems, respiratory problems, and local injection site pain (Dodick et al., 2010).

Imaging modalities used to perform procedure

Image guidance is not typically used while performing this procedure.

Type of medications used

Onabotulinum toxin A.

Sedations used

This procedure is not typically done with sedation.

Length of time for the procedure

Thirty minutes to 1 hour.

Expected postprocedural care

Monitor for any of the aforementioned side effects.

Frequency of having this procedure

This procedure may be done every 12 weeks for 2 years (Blumenfeld, Stark, Freeman, Orejudos, & Manack Adams, 2018).

Ways of documentation of efficacy

Documentation of treatment outcome can be done via (1) headache frequency, (2) headache length, (3) the Headache Impact Test-6 scores, and (4) analgesic intake (Szok, Csáti, Vécsei, & Tajti, 2015).

Malignant Pain

Each year, approximately 1.5 million people in the United States are diagnosed with cancer (American Cancer Society, 2013). Patients may experience cancer-related pain from tumor burden because of location, growth, or compression and displacement of the surrounding structures. Patients may also have pain related to treatments, including chemotherapy, radiation, and surgery. Identifying patients who would benefit from interventional procedures can help palliate and relieve the suffering from pain that these patients may have.

Palliative Radiation Therapy

Introduction

External beam radiation therapy (EBRT) and stereotactic body radiation therapy (SBRT) are palliative treatment options for cancer patients with bone metastases. The most common bone metastases arise from breast, prostate, and bone cancers, accounting for 80% of all cases (Falkmer, Järhult, Wersäll, & Cavallin-Ståhl, 2003). Bone metastases can disrupt nerve fibers in the periosteum, which can result in pain. Radiation acts by destroying tumor cells and decreasing bone mass effect.

> ▶ **KEY POINT**
>
> EBRT and SBRT aim to control pain, preserve function, stabilize bone, prevent fractures, and manage local tumors.

Of note, other options for bony metastases treatment include analgesics, systemic therapy (such as bisphosphonates, denosumab), chemotherapy, and/or surgery (Cai, Nickman, & Gaffney, 2013; Pin et al., 2018).

Clinical features

Bony metastases can produce skeletal or neuropathic pain (Falkmer et al., 2003). The character and intensity of pain vary, ranging from intermittent to frequent and dull to severe. The pain may refer to other regions of the body. Pain may be worse at night and at times improves with physical activity (Cai et al., 2013).

Physical examination findings

May vary depending on the location and/or number of metastases. Patients may present with signs or symptoms of hypercalcemia, nerve root involvement, fractures, and/or spinal cord compression (Falkmer et al., 2003).

Interventional procedure type

Palliative radiation therapy is an outpatient interventional procedure.

Brief description of procedure

Specific areas of bone metastases are targeted by an imaging modality such as CT. A radiation machine then delivers targeted beams onto the areas of bone metastases. Although the radiation fractionation schemes have not been standardized, the two most common schedules of irradiation are 8 Gy in a single fraction and 30 Gy in 10 fractions. There are many intermediate options (Pin et al., 2018).

Contraindications

This is a palliative treatment for patients with a short life expectancy.

Risk/potential adverse effects

Potential adverse effects from this procedure are: an increase in bone pain after treatment, acute radiation toxicity, and many of the common side effects associated with radiation (Cai et al., 2013).

Imaging modalities used to perform procedure

The imaging modalities used for this procedure are CT, MRI, and stereotactic guidance.

Type of medications

This is a radiation treatment.

Sedations used

Sedation is not typically used but this is at the discretion of the patient and provider.

Length of time for the procedure

The duration of the procedure varies mainly depending on the radiation fractionation and scheduling.

Expected postprocedural care

Typical postprocedural restrictions/limitations include: (1) avoidance of driving and (2) avoidance of strenuous activity following procedure. The patient should be closely monitored for worsening of pain and signs of infection. Immediate medical help should be sought if patient experiences sudden-onset weakness or loss of bowel/bladder function following procedure.

Frequency of having this procedure

Radiation treatment often causes long-lasting pain relief without need to repeat the procedure in 45% of patients (Hayashi, Hoshi, Iida, & Kajiura, 1999). There are no clear guidelines as to when should patients receive repeat treatment for peripheral bone metastases (Lutz et al., 2011).

Ways of documentation of efficacy

Documentation of treatment outcome can be done via (1) visual analog pain scale, (2) reduction of analgesic use, (3) Functional Assessment of Cancer Therapy quality of life measurement in patients with bone pain, and (4) the Edmonton Symptom Assessment System (Cai et al., 2013).

TABLE 9–1. Current Procedural Terminology (CPT) Codes

Procedure	Corresponding CPT Codes
Interlaminar (with fluoroscopic imaging)	
Interlaminar—cervical or thoracic	62321
Interlaminar—lumbar or sacral (caudal)	62323
Transforaminal (with fluoroscopic imaging)	
Transforaminal—cervical or thoracic (first level)	64479
Transforaminal—cervical or thoracic (each additional level)	64480
Transforaminal—lumbar or sacral (first level)	64483
Transforaminal—lumbar or sacral (each additional level)	64484
Intraarticular joint or medial branch block	
Intraarticular joint or medial branch block (MBB)—cervical or thoracic (first level)	64490
Intraarticular joint or medial branch block (MBB)—cervical or thoracic (second level)	64491
Intraarticular joint or medial branch block (MBB)—cervical or thoracic (third level)	64492
Intraarticular joint or medial branch block (MBB)—lumbar or sacral (first level)	64493
Intraarticular joint or medial branch block (MBB)—lumbar or sacral (second level)	64494
Intraarticular joint or medial branch block (MBB)—lumbar or sacral (third level)	64495
Radiofrequency ablation	
Radiofrequency ablation (RFA)—cervical or thoracic (first joint)	64633
Radiofrequency ablation (RFA)—cervical or thoracic (each additional joint)	64634
Radiofrequency ablation (RFA)—lumbar or sacral (first joint)	64635
Radiofrequency ablation (RFA)—lumbar or sacral (each additional joint)	64636
Sacroiliac joint procedures	
Sacroiliac joint (SIJ) without fluoroscopy	20552 (billed as a trigger point injection)
Sacroiliac joint (SIJ) with fluoroscopy	27096
Sacral lateral branch blocks	64450
Spinal cord stimulator procedures	
Trial procedure	
Percutaneous implant of electrode array	63650 (includes 10-day global)

Implantation of spinal cord stimulator, percutaneous leads, and generator	
Percutaneous implant of electrode array	63650 (includes 10-day global)
Insertion or replacement of pulse generator	63685 (includes 10-day global)
Implantation of spinal cord stimulator, paddle leads, and generator	
Laminectomy for implant of neurostimulator electrode, paddle	63655 (includes 90-day global)
Insertion or replacement of pulse generator	63685 (includes 10-day global)
Removal of leads/generator (explant)	
Removal of spinal neurostimulator percutaneous array(s)	63661 (includes 10-day global)
Removal of spinal neurostimulator paddle electrode	63662 (includes 90-day global)
Removal of pulse generator	63688 (includes 10-day global)
Reservoir/pump implantation	
Implantation or replacement of device for intrathecal or epidural drug infusion; a subcutaneous reservoir (10 days global)	62360
Implantation or replacement of device for intrathecal or epidural drug infusion; a nonprogrammable pump (10 days global)	62361
Implantation or replacement of device for intrathecal or epidural drug infusion; programmable pump, including preparation of pump, with or without programming (10 days global)	62362
Catheter implantation	
Implantation, revision, or repositioning of tunneled intrathecal or epidural catheter, for long-term medication administration via an external pump or implantable reservoir/infusion pump; without laminectomy (10 days global)	62350
Implantation, revision, or repositioning of tunneled intrathecal or epidural catheter, for long-term medication administration via an external pump or implantable reservoir/infusion pump; with laminectomy (90 days global)	62351
Refilling and maintenance of reservoir or pump without reprogramming	
Refilling and maintenance of implantable pump or reservoir for drug delivery, spinal (intrathecal, epidural) or brain (intraventricular), includes electronic analysis of pump when performed	95990
Refilling and maintenance of implantable pump or reservoir for drug delivery, spinal (intrathecal, epidural) or brain (intraventricular), includes electronic analysis of pump when performed; requiring the skill of a physician or other qualified healthcare professional	95991

(continued)

TABLE 9–1. Procedural CPT Codes (*continued*)

Procedure	Corresponding CPT Codes
Diskogram/diskography	
Diskogram/diskography—cervical/thoracic (each disk)	62291
Supervision and interpretation of fluoroscopy—cervical/thoracic (each disk)	72285
Diskogram/diskography—lumbar (each disk)	62290
Supervision and interpretation of fluoroscopy—lumbar (each disk)	72295
Nerve block	
Axillary nerve block	64417
Suprascapular nerve block	64418
Carpal tunnel block	20526
Intercostal nerve block (single)	64420
Intercostal nerve block (multiple)	64421
Ilioinguinal and iliohypogastric nerve block	64425
Pudendal nerve block	64430
Sciatic nerve block	64445
Plantar common digital nerve block	64455
Trigeminal nerve block (any branch)	64400
Other peripheral nerve block	64450
Unlisted procedure	64999
Sympathetically mediated blocks	
Stellate ganglion (cervical sympathetic)	64510
Thoracic or lumbar paravertebral sympathetic or ganglion impar block	64520
Orthopedic injections	
Major joint/bursa (knee, hip, shoulder, trochanteric bursa, subacromial bursa, pes anserine bursa)	20610
Intermediate joint/bursa (temporomandibular, acromioclavicular, wrist, elbow, ankle, olecranon bursa)	20605
Major joint/bursa (knee, hip, shoulder, trochanteric bursa, subacromial bursa, pes anserine bursa)	20610
Minor joint/bursa (fingers [proximal interphalangeal, distal interphalangeal], toes)	20600

Trigger point injections	
Injection(s); single or multiple trigger point(s), 1 or 2 muscle(s)	20552
Injection(s); single or multiple trigger point(s), 3 or more muscles	20553
Chemo denervation	
Botulinum toxin type A—Botox, Dysport (per unit)	J0585
Botulinum toxin type B—Myobloc (per 100 units)	J0587
Needle electromyography in conjunction with chemodenervation	95874
Chemodenervation of muscles in the neck (spasmodic torticollis)	64616
Chemodenervation of muscles of the trunk and/or extremity (cerebral palsy, dystonia, multiple sclerosis)	64614
Chemodenervation of muscles innervated by facial, trigeminal, cervical spinal and accessory nerves, bilateral (chronic migraine)	64615

REFERENCES

Adler, R. S., & Sofka, C. M. (2003). Percutaneous ultrasound-guided injections in the musculoskeletal system. *Ultrasound Quarterly, 19*(1), 3–12.

Alexander, C. E., & Dulebohn, S. C. (2018). Lumbar sympathetic block [Updated 2017 Nov 5]. In StatPearls [Internet]. Treasure Island, FL: StatPearls Publishing.

Allegri, M., Montella, S., Salici, F., Valente, A., Marchesini, M., Compagnone, C., . . . Fanelli, G. (2016). Mechanisms of low back pain: A guide for diagnosis and therapy. *F1000Res, 5.*

American Cancer Society. (2013). Cancer Facts and Figures 2013. http://www cancer.org/research/cancerfacrsfigures/cancerfactsfigures/cancer-facts-figures-2013

Artner, J., Cakir, B., Reichel, H., & Lattig, F. (2012). Radiation dose reduction in CT-guided sacroiliac joint injections to levels of pulsed fluoroscopy: A comparative study with technical considerations. *Journal of Pain Research, 5,* 265–269. doi:10.2147/JPR.S34429

Ayhan, E., Kesmezacar, H., & Akgun, I. (2014). Intraarticular injections (corticosteroid, hyaluronic acid, platelet rich plasma) for the knee osteoarthritis. *World Journal of Orthopedics, 5,* 351–361.

Baig, S., Moon, J. Y., & Shankar, H. (2017). Review of sympathetic blocks: Anatomy, sonoanatomy, evidence, and techniques. *Regional Anesthesia and Pain Medicine, 42*(3), 377–391. doi:10.1097/AAP.0000000000000591

Barolat, G., Oakley, J., Law, J., North, R. B., Ketcik, B., & Sharan, A. (2001). Epidural spinal cord stimulation with a multiple electrode paddle lead is effective in treating low back pain. *Neuromodulation, 4*(2), 59–66.

Ben-Haim, S., Mirzadeh, Z., & Rosenberg, W. S. (2018). Deep brain stimulation for intractable neuropathic facial pain. *Neurosurgical Focus, 45*(2), E15. doi:10.3171/2018.5.FOCUS18160

Blumenfeld, A. M., Stark, R. J., Freeman, M. C., Orejudos, A., & Manack Adams, A. (2018). Long-term study of the efficacy and safety of Onabotulinum toxin A for the prevention of chronic migraine: COMPEL study. *Journal of Headache and Pain, 19*(1), 13. doi:10.1186/s10194-018-0840-8

Boccard, S. G., Pereira, E. A., & Aziz, T. Z. (2015). Deep brain stimulation for chronic pain. *Journal of Clinical Neuroscience, 22*(10), 1537–15843. doi:10.1016/j.jocn.2015.04.005

Borg-Stein, J., & Iaccarino, M. A. (2014). Myofascial pain syndrome treatments. *Physical Medicine and Rehabilitation Clinics of North America, 25*(2), 357–374. doi:10.1016/j.pmr.2014.01.012

Boswell, M., Trescot, A. M., Datta, S., Schultz, D. M., Hansen, H. C., Abdi, S., . . . American Society of Interventional Pain Physicians. (2007). Interventional techniques: Evidence-based practice guidelines in the management of chronic spinal pain. *Pain Physician, 10,* 7–111.

Bottros, M. M., & Christo, P. J. (2014). Current perspectives on intrathecal drug delivery. *Journal of Pain Research, 7,* 615–626. doi:10.2147/JPR.S37591

Bruehl, S. (2015). Complex regional pain syndrome. *BMJ, 351,* h2730.

Buchanan, B. K., & Dulebohn, S. C. (2018). Radial nerve entrapment. [Updated 2017 May 31]. In StatPearls [Internet]. Treasure Island, FL: StatPearls Publishing. Retrieved from https://www.ncbi.nlm.nih.gov/books/NBK431097/

Burton, C. (1975). Dorsal column stimulation: Optimization of application. *Surgical Neurology, 4,* 171–176.

Cai, B., Nickman, N. A., & Gaffney, D. K. (2013). The role of palliative external beam radiation therapy in boney metastases pain management. *Journal of Pain and Palliative Care Pharmacotherapy, 27*(1), 28–34. doi:10.3109/15360288.2012.757267

Carroll, I., Clark, J. D., & Mackey, S. (2009). Sympathetic block with botulinum toxin to treat complex regional pain syndrome. *Annals of Neurology, 65*(3), 348–351.

Cass, S. P. (2015). Piriformis syndrome: A cause of nondiscogenic sciatica. *Current Sports Medicine Reports, 14*(1), 41–44. doi:10.1249/JSR.0000000000000110

Cass, S. P. (2016). Ultrasound-guided nerve hydro dissection: What is it? A review of the literature. *Current Sports Medicine Reports, 15,* 20–22.

Chakravarthy, K., Nava, A., Christo, P. J., & Williams, K. (2016). Review of recent advances in peripheral nerve stimulation (PNS). *Current Pain and Headache Reports, 20*(11), 60.

Chan, C. W., & Peng, P. (2011). Failed back surgery syndrome. *Pain Medicine, 12*(4), 577–606. doi:10.1111/j.1526-4637.2011.01089.x

Chan, I., Brown, A. R., Park, K., & Winfree, C. J. (2010). Ultrasound-guided, percutaneous peripheral nerve stimulation: Technical note. *Neurosurgery, 67*(3 Suppl Operative), ons136–ons139.

Chang, A., & White, B. A. (2017). Peripheral nerve blocks. [Updated 2017 Oct 6]. In StatPearls [Internet]. Treasure Island, FL: StatPearls Publishing. Retrieved from https://www.ncbi.nlm.nih.gov/books/NBK459210/

Chen, M. J. L., Lew, H. L., Hsu, T.-C., Tsai, W.-C., Lin, W.-C., Tang, S. F. T., . . . Chen, C. P. (2006). Ultrasound-guided shoulder injections in the treatment of subacromial bursitis. *American Journal of Physical Medicine & Rehabilitation, 85*(1), 31–35. doi:10.1097/01.phm.0000184158.85689.5e

Cheng, J., & Abdi, S. (2007). Complications of joint, tendon, and muscle injections. *Techniques in Regional Anesthesia and Pain Management, 11*(3), 141–147. doi:10.1053/j.trap.2007.05.006

Cheng, O. T., Souzdalnitski, D., Vrooman, B., & Cheng, J. (2012). Evidence-based knee injections for the management of arthritis. *Pain Medicine, 13*(6), 740–753. doi:10.1111/j.1526-4637.2012.01394.x

Chu, J. (1995). Dry needling (intramuscular stimulation) in myofascial pain related to lumbar radiculopathy. *European Journal of Physical Medicine and Rehabilitation, 5,* 106–121.

Cruccu, G., Finnerup, N. B., Jensen, T. S., Scholz, J., Sindou, M., Svensson, P., . . . Nurmikko, T. (2016). Trigeminal neuralgia: New classification and diagnostic grading for practice and research. *Neurology, 87,* 220–228.

Cruccu, G., Gronseth, G., Alksne, J., Argoff, C., Brainin, M., Burchiel, K., . . . European Federation of Neurological Society. (2008). AAN-EFNS guidelines on trigeminal neuralgia management. *European Journal of Neurology, 15*, 1013–1028. doi:10.1111/j.1468-1331.2008. 02185.x

Daniels, E. W., Cole, D., Jacobs, B., & Phillips, S. F. (2018). Existing evidence on ultrasound-guided injections in sports medicine. *Orthopedic Journal of Sports Medicine, 6*(2), 2325967118756576.

Dawson, J., Linsell, L., Doll, H., Zondervan, K., Rose, P., Carr, A., . . . Fitzpatrick, R. (2005). Assessment of the Lequesne index of severity for osteoarthritis of the hip in an elderly population. *Osteo Arthritis and Cartilage, 13*, 854–860.

Deer, T., Mekhail, N., Provenzano, D., Pope, J., Krames, E., Thomson, S., . . . Neuromodulation Appropriateness Consensus Committee. (2014). The appropriate use of neurostimulation: Avoidance and treatment of complications of neurostimulation therapies for the treatment of chronic pain. Neuromodulation appropriateness consensus committee. *Neuromodulation, 17*(6), 571–597.

Dodick, D. W., Turkel, C. C., DeGryse, R. E., Aurora, S. K., Silberstein, S. D., Lipton, R. B., . . . PREEMPT chronic migraine study group. (2010). Onabotulinum toxin A for treatment of chronic migraine: Pooled results from the double-blind, randomized, placebo-controlled phases of the PREEMPT clinical program. *Headache, 50*, 921–936.

Duarte, R., Raphael, J., & Eldabe, S. (2016). Intrathecal drug delivery for the management of pain and spasticity in adults: An executive summary of the British Pain Society's recommendations for best clinical practice. *British Journal of Pain, 10*, 67–69.

Duarte, R., Raphael, J., Sparkes, E., Southall, J., Lemarchand, K., & Ashford, R. (2011). Long-term intrathecal drug administration for chronic nonmalignant pain. *Journal of Neurosurgical Anesthesiology, 24*, 63–70.

Dussault, R., Kaplan, P., & Anderson, M. (2000). Fluoroscopy-guided sacroiliac joint injections. *Radiology, 214*, 273–277.

Ehlers, L., Jensen, J. M., & Bendtsen, T. F. (2012). Cost-effectiveness of ultrasound vs nerve stimulation guidance for continuous sciatic nerve block. *British Journal of Anaesthesia, 109*, 804–808.

Eldabe, S., Duarte, R., Raphael, J., Thomson, S., & Bojanic, S. (2015). *Intrathecal drug delivery for the management of pain and spasticity in adults; recommendations for best clinical practice*. London: British Pain Society.

Espejo-Antúnez, L., Tejeda, J. F., Albornoz-Cabello, M., Rodríguez-Mansilla, J., de la Cruz-Torres, B., Ribeiro, F., & Silva, A. G. (2017). Dry needling in the management of myofascial trigger points: A systematic review of randomized controlled trials. *Complementary Therapies in Medicine, 33*, 46–57. doi:10.1016/j.ctim.2017.06.003

Falkmer, U., Järhult, J., Wersäll, P., & Cavallin-Ståhl, E. (2003). A systematic overview of radiation therapy effects in skeletal metastases. *Acta Oncologica, 42*(5–6), 620–633.

Falowski, S. M. (2015). Deep brain stimulation for chronic pain. *Current Pain and Headache Reports, 19*(7), 27. doi:10.1007/s11916-015-0504-1

Finoff, J. T., Hurdle, M. F., & Smith, J. (2008). Accuracy of ultrasound-guided versus fluoroscopically guided contrast-controlled piriformis injections. A cadaveric study. *Journal of Ultrasound in Medicine, 27*, 1157–1163.

Forst, S. L., Wheeler, M. T., Fortin, J. D., & Vilensky, J. A. (2006). (2007). The sacroiliac joint: Anatomy, physiology and clinical significance. *Pain Physician, 9*(1), 61–67.

Freedman, M., Greis, A. C., Marino, L., Sinha, A. N., & Henstenburg, J. (2014). Complex regional pain syndrome: Diagnosis and treatment. *Physical Medicine and Rehabilitation Clinics of North America, 25*(2), 291–303. doi:10.1016/j.pmr.2014.01.003

Friedrich, J. M., & Harrast, M. A. (2010). Lumbar epidural steroid injections: Indications, contraindications, risks, and benefits. *Current Sports Medicine Reports, 9*(1), 43–49. doi:10.1249/JSR.0b013e3181caa7fc

Gadsen, J. (2013, October). Local anesthetics: Clinical pharmacology and rational selection. The New York School of Regional Anesthesia website. Retrieved from http://www.nysora.com/regional-anesthesia/foundations-of-ra/3492-local-anesthetics-clinical-pharmacology-and-rational-selection.html

Garmon, E. H., & O'Rourke , M. C. (2018). Anesthesia, Nerve Block. [Updated 2017]. In: StatPearls [Internet]. Treasure Island (FL): StatPearls Publishing. Retrieved from https://www.ncbi.nlm.nih.gov/books/NBK431109/

Gellhorn, A. C., Katz, J. N., & Suri, P. (2013). Osteoarthritis of the spine: The facet joints. *Nature Reviews Rheumatology, 9*(4), 216–224. doi:10.1038/nrrheum.2012.199

Goroszeniuk, T., & Pang, D. (2014). Peripheral neuromodulation: A review. *Current Pain and Headache Reports, 18*(5), 412. doi:10.1007/s11916-014-0412-9

Groiss, S. J., Wojtecki, L., Südmeyer, M., & Schnitzler, A. (2009). Deep brain stimulation in Parkinson's disease. *Therapeutic Advances in Neurological Disorders, 2*(6), 20–28. doi:10.1177/1756285609339382

Hayashi, S., Hoshi, H., Iida, T., & Kajiura, Y. (1999). Multi-fractionated wide-field radiation therapy for palliation of multiple symptomatic bone metastases from solid tumors. *Radiation Medicine, 17*(6), 411–416.

Headache Classification Committee of the International Headache Society. (2013). The international classification of headache disorders, 3rd edition (beta version). *Cephalalgia, 33*, 629–808.

Huber, S., & Vaglienti, R. (2000). Spinal cord stimulation in severe, inoperable, peripheral vascular disease. *Neuromodulation, 3*, 131–143.

Jankovic, D., Peng, P., & van Zundert, A. (2013). Brief review: Piriformis syndrome: Etiology, diagnosis and management. *Canadian Journal of Anaesthesia, 60*, 1003Y1012.

Joshi, G., Gandhi, K., Shah, N., Gadsden, J., & Corman, S. L. (2016). Peripheral nerve blocks in the management of postoperative pain: Challenges and opportunities. *Journal of Clinical Anesthesia, 35*, 524–529.

Jung, J. H., Kim, H. I., Shin, D. A., Shin, D. G., Lee, J. O., Kim, H. J., & Chung, J. H. (2007). Usefulness of pain distribution pattern assessment in decision-making for the patients with lumbar zygapophyseal and sacroiliac joint arthropathy. *Journal of Korean Medical Science, 22*, 1048–1054.

Jüni, P., Hari, R., Rutjes, A. W. S., Fischer, R., Silletta, M. G., Reichenbach, S., & da Costa, B. R. (2015). Intra-articular corticosteroid for knee osteoarthritis. *Cochrane Database System Review*, (Issue 10); Art. No.: CD005328. doi:10.1002/14651858.CD005328.pub3

Kietrys, D. M., Palombaro, K. M., Azzaretto, E., Hubler, R., Schaller, B., Schlussel, J. M., & Tucker, M. (2013). Effectiveness of dry needling for upper-quarter myofascial pain: A systematic review and meta-analysis. *The Journal of Orthopaedic and Sports Physical Therapy, 43*(9), 620–634. doi:10.2519/jospt.2013.4668

Kirschner, J. S., Foye, P. M., & Cole, J. L. (2009). Piriformis syndrome, diagnosis and treatment. *Muscle & Nerve, 40*(1), 10–18. doi:10.1002/mus.21318

Knight, K. H., Brand, F. M., Mchaourab, A. S., & Veneziano, G. (2007). Implantable intrathecal pumps for chronic pain: Highlights and updates. *Croatian Medical Journal, 48*, 22–34.

Kowalska, B., & Sudoł-Szopińska, I. (2012). Ultrasound assessment on selected peripheral nerve pathologies. Part I: Entrapment neuropathies of the upper limb—Excluding carpal tunnel syndrome. *Journal of Ultrasonography, 12*, 307–318.

Kreis, P. G., & Fischman, S. A. (2009). *Spinal cord stimulation: Percutaneous implantation techniques*. New York: Oxford University Press.

Kumar, S., Rastogi, S., Mahendra, P., Bansal, M., & Chandra, L. (2013). Pain in trigeminal neuralgia: Neurophysiology and measurement: A comprehensive review. *Journal of Medicine and Life, 15*, 383–388.

Lam, S., Reeves, K. D., & Cheng, A. L. (2017). Transition from deep regional blocks toward deep nerve hydro dissection in the upper body and torso: Method description and results from a retrospective chart review of the analgesic effect of 5% dextrose water as the primary hydro dissection Injectate to enhance safety. *BioMed Research International, 2017,* 7920438. doi:10.1155/2017/7920438

Latif, O. A., Nedeljkovic, S. S., & Stevenson, L. W. (2001). Spinal cord stimulation for chronic intractable angina: A unified pectoris unified theory on its mechanism. *Clinical Cardiology, 24,* 533–541.

Leak, W. D. (2006). Epidural steroid injections. In M. V. Boswell & B. E. Cole (Eds.), *Weiner's pain management* (7th ed., pp. 289–295). Boca Raton, FL: CRC Press.

Lin, E., Choi, J., & Hadzic, A. (2013). Peripheral nerve blocks for outpatient surgery: Evidence-based indications. *Current Opinions in Anesthesiology, 26,* 467.

Liow, Y., Wang, W., & Loh, V. W. K. (2017). Outpatient management of knee osteoarthritis. *Singapore Medical Journal, 58*(10), 580–584. doi:10.11622/smedj.2017097

Lutz, S., Berk, L., Chang, E., Hahn, C., Hoskin, P., Howell, D., . . . American Society for Radiation Oncology (ASTRO). (2011). Palliative radiotherapy for bone metastases: An ASTRO evidence-based guideline. *International Journal of Radiation Oncology, Biology, Physics, 79*(4), 965–976.

Maarbjerg, S., Di Stefano, G., Bendtsen, L., & Cruccu, G. (2017). Trigeminal neuralgia—Diagnosis and treatment. *Cephalalgia, 37,* 33310241668728. doi:10.1177/0333102416687280

Majlesi, J., & Unalan, H. (2010). Effect of treatment on trigger points. *Current Pain and Headache Reports, 14*(5), 353–360.

Maleki, J., LeBel, A. A., Bennett, G. J., & Schwartzman, R. J. (2000). Patterns of spread in complex regional pain syndrome, type I (reflex sympathetic dystrophy). *Pain, 88*(3), 259–266.

Mallow, M., & Nazarian, L. N. (2014). Greater trochanteric pain syndrome diagnosis and treatment. *Physical Medicine and Rehabilitation Clinics of North America, 25*(2), 279–289. doi:10.1016/j.pmr.2014.01.009

Manchikanti, L., Damron, K. S., Rivera, J. J., McManus, C. D., Jackson, S. D., Barnhill, R. C., & Martin, J. C. (2004). Evaluation of the effect of sedation as a confounding factor in the diagnostic validity of lumbar facet joint pain: A prospective, randomized, double-blind, placebo-controlled evaluation. *Pain Physician, 7*(4), 411–417.

Manchikanti, L., Hirsch, J. A., Falco, F. J., & Boswell, M. V. (2016). Management of lumbar zygapophyseal (facet) joint pain. *World Journal of Orthopedics, 7*(5), 315–337. doi:10.5312/wjo. v7. i5.315

Manchikanti, L., Kaye, A. D., Boswell, M. V., Bakshi, S., Gharibo, C. G., Grami, V., . . . Hirsch, J. A. (2015). A systematic review and best evidence synthesis of the effectiveness of therapeutic facet joint interventions in managing chronic spinal pain. *Pain Physician, 18*(4), E535–E582.

Manchikanti, L., Staats, P. S., Singh, V., Schultz, D. M., Vilims, B. D., Jasper, J. F., . . . Feler, C. A. (2003). Evidence-based practice guidelines for interventional techniques in the management of chronic spinal pain. *Pain Physician, 6*(1), 3–81.

Maricar, N., Parkes, M. J., Callaghan, M. J., Felson, D. T., & O'Neill, T. W. (2013). Where and how to inject the knee—A systematic review. *Seminars in Arthritis and Rheumatism, 43*(2), 195–203. doi:10.1016/j.semarthrit.2013.04.010

Mekhail, N. A., Mathews, M., Nageeb, F., Guirguis, M., Mekhail, M. N., & Cheng, J. (2011). Retrospective review of 707 cases of spinal cord stimulation: Indications and complications. *Pain Practice, 11*(2), 148–153. doi:10.1111/j.1533-2500.2010.00407.x

Meyer, P., Lintingre, P.-F., Pesquer, L., Poussange, N., Silvestre, A., & Dallaudière, B. (2018). The median nerve at the carpal tunnel . . . and elsewhere. *Journal of the Belgian Society of Radiology, 102*(1), 17. doi:10.5334/jbsr.1354

Michel, F., Decavel, P., Toussirot, E., Tatu, L., Aleton, E., Monnier, G., . . . Parratte, B. (2013). The piriformis muscle syndrome: An exploration of anatomical context, pathophysiological hypotheses and diagnostic criteria. *Annals of Physical and Rehabilitation Medicine, 56*(4), 300–311. doi:10.1016/j.rehab.2013.03.006

Molini, L., Mariacher, S., & Bianchi, S. (2012). US guided corticosteroid injection into the subacromial-subdeltoid bursa: Technique and approach. *Journal of Ultrasound, 15*, 61–68.

Monseau, A. J., & Nizran, P. S. (2013). Common injections in musculoskeletal medicine. *Primary Care, 40*(4), 987–1000, ix-x. doi:10.1016/j.pop.2013.08.012

Moskovitz, J. B., & Sabatino, F. (2013). Regional nerve blocks of the face. *Emergency Medicine Clinics of North America, 31*(2), 517–527.

Oakley, J., & Prager, J. (2002). Spinal cord stimulation: Mechanism of action. *Spine, 22*, 2574–2583.

Pang, N., Mahajan, M., & Fishmann, S. (2005). *Pain medicine and management: Just the facts* (1st ed., pp. 336–341). New York: McGraw-Hill.

Patel, K., & Upadhyayula, S. (2018). Epidural steroid injections. [Updated 2017 Nov 22]. In StatPearls [Internet]. Treasure Island, FL: StatPearls Publishing. Retrieved from https://www.ncbi.nlm.nih.gov/books/NBK470189/

Patel, V. B., Wasserman, R., & Imani, F. (2015). Interventional therapies for chronic low Back Pain: A focused review (efficacy and outcomes). *Anesthesiology in Pain Medicine, 5*(4), e29716. doi:10.5812/aapm.29716

Paterson, K. L., Hunter, D. J., Metcalf, B. R., Eyles, J., Duong, V., Kazsa, J., . . . Bennell, K. L. (2018). Efficacy of intra-articular injections of platelet-rich plasma as a symptom- and disease-modifying treatment for knee osteoarthritis—The RESTORE trial protocol. *BMC Musculoskeletal Disorders, 19*(272). doi:10.1186/s12891-018-2205-5

Payne, J. M. (2016). Ultrasound-guided hip procedures. *Physical Medicine and Rehabilitation Clinics of North America, 27*(3), 607–629. doi:10.1016/j.pmr.2016.04.004

Petersen, E. A., & Slavin, K. V. (2014). Peripheral nerve/field stimulation for chronic pain. *Neurosurgery Clinics of North America, 25*(4), 789–797. doi:10.1016/j.nec.2014.07.003

Pin, Y., Paix, A., Le Fèvre, C., Antoni, D., Blondet, C., & Noël, G. (2018). A systematic review of palliative bone radiotherapy based on pain relief and retreatment rates. *Critical Reviews in Oncology/Hematology, 123*, 132–137. doi:10.1016/j.critrevonc.2018.01.006

Raj, M. A., & Dulebohn, S. C. (2018). Pain, sacroiliac joint. [Updated 2017 Nov 8]. In: StatPearls [Internet]. Treasure Island, FL: StatPearls Publishing. Retrieved from https://www.ncbi.nlm.nih.gov/books/NBK470299/

Rowlingson, J. (2005). *Pain medicine and management: Just the facts* (1st ed., pp. 289–295). New York: McGraw-Hill.

Scholten, P. M., Patel, S. I., Christos, P. J., & Singh, J. R. (2015). Short-term efficacy of Sacroiliac joint corticosteroid injection based on arthrographic contrast patterns. *PM & R: The Journal of Injury, Function, and Rehabilitation, 7*(4), 385–391.

Schwarzer, A. C., Aprill, C. N., Derby, R., Fortin, J., Kine, G., & Bogduk, N. (1994). The relative contributions of the disc and zygapophyseal joint in chronic low back pain. *Spine (Phila Pa 1976), 19*(7), 801–806.

Shah, J. P., Thaker, N., Heimur, J., Aredo, J. V., Sikdar, S., & Gerber, L. H. (2015). Myofascial trigger points then and now: A historical and scientific perspective. *PM & R: The Journal of Injury, Function, and Rehabilitation, 7*(7), 746–761. doi:10.1016/j.pmrj.2015.01.024

Simon, J., McAuliffe, M., Shamim, F., Vuong, N., & Tahaei, A. (2014). Discogenic low back pain. *Physical Medicine and Rehabilitation Clinics of North America, 25*(2), 305–317. doi:10.1016/j.pmr.2014.01.006

Simons, D. G., Travell, J. G., & Travell, S. L. S. (1999). *Simons' myofascial pain and dysfunction: The trigger point manual* (2nd ed., pp. 94–173). Baltimore: Williams & Wilkins.

Sjm.com. (2018). Recovering after SCS and neurostimulation surgery | St. Jude Medical. [online] Retrieved from https://www.sjm.com/en/patients/chronic-pain/getting-a-system/recovering-after-the-procedure?clset=af584191-45c9-4201-8740-5409f4cf8bdd%3ab20716c1-c2a6-4e4c-844b-d0dd6899eb3a

Smith, J., Hurdle, M. F., Locketz, A. J., & Wisniewski, S. J. (2006). Ultrasound-guided piriformis injection: Technique description and verification. *Archives of Physical Medicine and Rehabilitation, 87*(12), 1664–1667.

Srejic, U., Calvillo, O., & Kabakibou, K. (1999). Viscosupplementation: A new concept in the treatment of sacroiliac joint syndrome: A preliminary report of four cases. *Regional Anesthesia and Pain Medicine, 24,* 84–88.

Swagerty, D. L., Jr., & Hellinger, D. (2001). Radiographic assessment of osteoarthritis. *American Family Physician, 64,* 279–286.

Szadek, K. M., van der Wurff, P., van Tulder, M. W., Zuurmond, W. W., & Perez, R. S. (2008). Diagnostic validity of criteria for sacroiliac joint pain: A systematic review. *The Journal of Pain, 10*(4), 354–368.

Szok, D., Csáti, A., Vécsei, L., & Tajti, J. (2015). Treatment of chronic migraine with Onabotulinum toxin A: Mode of action, efficacy and safety. *Toxins, 7*(7), 2659–2673. doi:10.3390/toxins7072659

Telli, H., Telli, S., & Topal, M. (2018). The validity and reliability of provocation tests in the diagnosis of Sacroiliac joint dysfunction. *Pain Physician, 21*(4), E367–E376.

Turesson, C., O'Fallon, W., Crowson, C., Gabriel, S., & Matteson, E. (2003). Extra-articular disease manifestations in rheumatoid arthritis: Incidence trends and risk factors over 46 years. *Annals of the Rheumatic Diseases, 62*(8), 722–727. doi:10.1136/ard.62.8.722

Wahal, C., Kumar, A., & Pyati, S. (2018). Advances in regional anaesthesia: A review of current practice, newer techniques and outcomes. *Indian Journal of Anaesthesia, 62,* 94–102.

Waldam, S. (2006). Sympathetic neural blockade in the evaluation and treatment of pain. In M. V. Boswell & B. E. Cole (Eds.), *Weiner's pain management* (7th ed., pp. 925–938). Boca Raton, FL: CRC Press.

Whitcup, S. M., Turkel, C. C., DeGryse, R. E., & Brin, M. F. (2014). Development of onabotulinum toxin A for chronic migraine. *Annals of the New York Academy of Sciences, 1329,* 67–80.

Zakrzewska, J. M., & McMillan, R. (2011). Trigeminal neuralgia: The diagnosis and management of this excruciating and poorly understood facial pain. *Postgraduate Medical Journal, 87,* 410–416.

CHAPTER 10

SURGICAL AND PROCEDURAL PAIN MANAGEMENT

Mallory Perry

Introduction

Adequate and appropriate pain management is a basic human right, as stated by the World Health Organization (WHO) and the International Association for the Study of Pain (Brennan, Carr, & Cousins, 2007). Postsurgical pain is unique and multivariate, requiring individualized care plans to ensure that the pain is treated and managed well. Unrelieved pain in the postoperative period may lead to negative sequalae including, but not limited to, increased rehabilitation postoperatively as well as persistent postoperative pain (PPP) development. The following chapter will outline postoperative pain, its assessment, management, and special considerations.

Postoperative Pain Physiology and Prevalence

The way in which pain is processed, and experienced, depends on inherent characteristics of the individual and the type of the procedure itself. To understand postoperative pain, the type of pain must first be understood. Nociceptive pain is the most common pain experienced by individuals and is generally the pain that is experienced postoperatively. As defined by the International Association for the Study of Pain (1994), nociceptive pain is defined as "pain that arises from actual or threatened damage to non-neural tissue and is due to the activation of nociceptors." Nociceptors are "high-threshold sensory receptors of the peripheral somatosensory nervous system, that [are] capable of transducing and encoding noxious stimuli." When there is an insult to tissue, such as with a surgical procedure, pain processing involves a feedback response as detailed in Figure 10-1. In addition to understanding the type of pain, distinction must be made concerning the classification of pain dependent on duration of symptoms, that is,

> ▶ **KEY POINT**
>
> Up to 85% of adults and 20% of children may experience a type of chronic pain, referred to as PPP (Macrae, 2001; Niraj & Rowbotham, 2011; Rabbitts, Fisher, Rosenbloom, & Palermo, 2017; Williams, Howard, & Liossi, 2017).

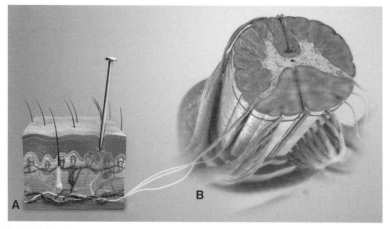

Figure 10–1. Nociception. A, A physical insult, in this case, a nail to soft tissue (i.e., skin), occurs causing actual and/or potential tissue damage. Nerve cells within the tissue are activated. B, Afferent neuronal impulses leave the site of injury and reach the spinal cord's dorsal horn. Here pain is transmitted and processed. Permission for use granted by Scientific Animations under Creative Commons license BY-SA 4.0 (https://creativecommons.org/licenses/by-sa/4.0/). Image can be found at http://www.scientificanimations.com/wiki-images

acute versus chronic. Acute pain is short in duration and generally resolves once the initial insult has healed. Contrarily, chronic pain lasts longer to heal than the initial insult, lasting months to years in duration. Acute postoperative pain is a fairly common and expected phenomenon.

PPP is defined as pain that lasts beyond the initial procedural insult, greater than 8 weeks (Macrae, 2001). Its prevalence depends on the type of procedure, with orthopedic procedures increasing this risk significantly. Moderate to severe postsurgical pain in the immediate postoperative pain period is a risk factor for PPP (Kehlet, Jensen, & Woolf, 2006; Perry, Starkweather, Baumbauer, & Young, 2018). For this reason, it is vital to ensure that healthcare providers are adequately assessing and managing postoperative pain throughout the perioperative period, including preoperative and postoperative, acute and chronic.

In understanding those who are at increased risk of PPP, a biopsychosocial approach should be taken when assessing patients preoperatively. In using this approach, the individual's entire being is considered. Table 10-1 outlines those who may be at increased risk for transitioning from acute to chronic pain states.

Postoperative Pain Assessment

Assessing pain throughout the perioperative period is vital to preventing long-term complications, including PPP. Relieving pain, while reducing the incidence of pharmacologic side effects, is of the utmost importance. Appropriate assessment of the pain both preoperatively and postoperatively will assist in ensuring that the pain trajectory is well managed. In adult populations, there are several assessment tools that may be used dependent upon the individual's cognitive function. As always, the gold

Table 10-1. Increased Postoperative Pain Risk Factors

Biopsychosocial	Pain catastrophizing, anxiety, a priori pain experiences, preoperative pain, etc. (Gatchel, Peng, Peters, Fuchs, & Turk, 2007; Gerbershagen et al., 2014; Logan & Rose, 2005)
Gender	Females have been reported to have increased postprocedural pain (Fillingim, King, Ribeiro-Dasilva, Rahim-Williams, & Riley, 2009; Gerbershagen et al., 2014)
Age	Elderly individuals are more sensitive to pain than younger patients, middle-aged and young adult (Gerbershagen et al., 2014; Wandner et al., 2012)
Socioeconomic status	Low socioeconomic status relates to decreased access to pain management services, leading to increased pain states (Feldman, Dong, Katz, Donnell-Fink, & Losina, 2015)
Genetic variation	Disease states such as sickle cell disease and inherent predisposition can influence an individual's perception, expression of pain, and overall sensitivity to stimuli (Chakravorty & Williams, 2015)

standard of pain assessment is patient self-report, and having a first-hand account of the patient's pain is vital. Choosing the correct scale is the initial point of assessment, done in conjunction with a comprehensive assessment. Conducting a pain interview using a pneumonic such as PQRSTU (Table 10-2) may be useful to ensure that the entire pain experience is captured and adequately assessed. Generally assessed on a numerical scale of 0 to 10, other instruments such as a visual analog scale may be used in those who are nonverbal. In children under 7 years of age, or unable to conceptualize the 0 to 10 concept, it may be helpful to utilize a visual scale such as Wong-Baker FACES pain rating scale (Wong-Baker Faces Foundation, 2016). If one is unable to provide a verbal account of pain, such as in the case of children or adults with neurocognitive impairment, it may be appropriate to use behavioral scales, such as the Faces, Legs, Arms, Crying, and Consolability (FLACC) scale (Merkel, Voepel-Lewis, Shayevitz, & Malviya, 1997). Though the gold standard is self-report, a proxy may be necessary in those who are unable to communicate (i.e., a caretaker or parent).

Table 10-2. PQRSTU Pain Interview

Provoke/palliative	What makes the pain better or worse?
Quality	What is the pain like (i.e., sharp, dull, stabbing)?
Radiation	Where else is the pain (i.e., referred pain)?
Severity	Quantification through developmentally appropriate pain scales
Timing	When did the pain begin?
Understanding	What does the pain mean for you? Quality of life?

The WHO Pain Ladder

Figure 10-2 outlines the WHO pain management ladder, providing a list of commonly used medications. It is important to note that this list is not inclusive of all medications and adjuvants. Initially created as a guide for those treating cancer pain, the WHO ladder has now been implicated for use in all types of pain, including postoperative pain (Gupta et al., 2010; Ventafridda, Saita, Ripamonti, & De Conno, 1985). The ladder differentiates mild, moderate, and severe pain states, with recommendations for the type of analgesic to be prescribed and subsequently administered. Each step builds upon each other as the pain persists. Step 1 involves the use of a nonopioid, step 2 may include a weak opioid in conjunction with a nonopioid, whereas step 3 escalates utilizing strong opioids with addition of nonopioids. At all stages of the ladder, an adjuvant and/or complementary alternative medicine (CAM) may be used. Considering the extensive nature of surgical procedures, it is not uncommon for pain management to begin at step 3, severe pain, in the immediate postoperative period and be titrated as appropriate to the patient's tolerance and pain level. Adequate titration of analgesics, dependent on the patient's pain, may improve long-term outcomes, such as decreased incidence of opioid dependence and withdrawal.

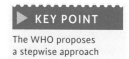

▶ **KEY POINT**

The WHO proposes a stepwise approach to managing pain in individuals (WHO, 1986).

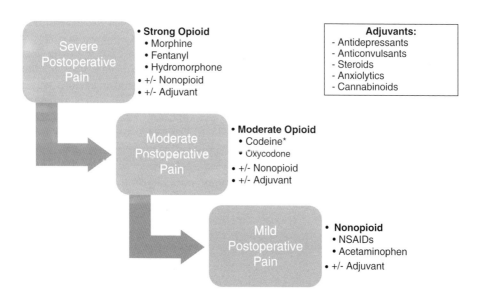

*Codeine should not be used routinely in children postoperatively, related to potentially toxic metabolites.

Figure 10–2. Analgesic ladder for postoperative pain. NSAID, nonsteroidal anti-inflammatory drug. Adapted from World Health Organization (1986).

▌Opioid Analgesia

Opioids are likely be the first-line analgesic choice considering the severe intensity of pain in the immediate postoperative period. Inherently, humans possess endogenous opioids and their respective receptors. Exogenous opioids, those that healthcare providers administer (i.e., morphine), work by binding to endogenous opioid receptors. In doing so, the opioid essentially alters pain modulation through the peripheral nervous system and central nervous system (CNS). There are several formularies of opioids, including oral, intravenous, transdermal, and rectal (Garimella & Cellini, 2013). The long-standing opioid of choice continues to be morphine, which is classified as a strong opioid. All other analgesics are compared to morphine via morphine equivalents (Pathan & Williams, 2012). Other strong opioids that may be comparative to morphine include fentanyl and hydromorphone (Table 10-3). These analgesics are synthetic derivatives of morphine, which make them more potent with shorter onset of action and half-lives (Garimella & Cellini, 2013).

Though opioids are very useful in managing severe postoperative pain, it is important to note their increased incidence of side effects. These side effects may include pruritus, opioid-induced constipation, opioid-induced hyperalgesia (OIH), and, most importantly, respiratory arrest. It is also important for providers to be aware of the risks of OIH. The rotation of opioids from different structural classes may also be helpful in this matter (Bottemiller, 2012). In addition, close monitoring of respiratory rate and depth is vital to ensuring the safety and efficacy of opioid administration. While administering morphine in the inpatient setting, sedation scales such as the Pasero Opioid-Induced Sedation Scale are useful in ensuring that the patient is tolerating the analgesia as well as providing recommendations for those who are not (Pasero, 2009). If the patient is deemed to be in respiratory depression or experiencing hypoxia, the opioid reversal agent is Naloxone, an opioid receptor antagonist.

In 2001, the Joint Commission saw an undertreatment of pain in individuals. In response, guidelines outlining pain assessment and reevaluation of the pain were created (Phillips, 2000). To facilitate change in practice of more thorough and frequent assessment and reassessment of pain, the Joint Commission referred to pain as the sixth vital sign. An unintended consequence of the focus on providing adequate treatment of pain was that the rate of opioid prescribing not only increased, but also precipitated the widespread fear of opioids, lack of consumer and prescriber education, inaccurate and inconsistent prescribing practices, as well as increased misuse

Table 10-3. Equianalgesic Chart of Strong Opioids Used for Postoperative Pain

	Oral (mg)	Intravenous or Intramuscular (mg)
Morphine	30	10
Fentanyl	N/A[*]	0.1
Hydromorphone	7.5	1.3

[*]Not indicated route for postoperative surgical procedure.

and abuse. Statistics from the current opioid epidemic both nationwide and at the state levels are enough to raise concern regarding opioid prescribing in the hospital setting. It is important to note that the majority of opioid use stems from opioids that have been legally prescribed and obtained. In 2015, there were 12.5 million people nationwide misusing prescription opioids, which subsequently cost the United States $78.5 billion (United States Department of Health and Human Services, 2017).

Patient-Controlled Analgesia

Depending on the patient's age, mental status, and cognitive function, the use of patient-controlled analgesia (PCA) may be beneficial in their treatment plan. PCA provides a way to secure intravenous or epidural analgesic medication at the bedside of the patient and the pump can be programmed to deliver continuous infusion or intermittent bolus dosing that is activated by the patient on a scheduled dosing scheme. Not only does a PCA afford patient autonomy but allows for continuous pain control. Generally, strong opioids, such as morphine, hydromorphone, and fentanyl, are used in PCA pumps. The modes in which PCA pumps can be set include continuous and demand or demand only. Lockout intervals should be appropriate and promote safe dosing while decreasing the negative side effects of opioids, such as sedation, cardiovascular collapse, hypoxia, and/or respiratory arrest. Adequate assessment of individuals who may be most appropriate for PCA analgesic is vital to ensuring its overall efficacy. PCA pumps are not appropriate for young children and/or those who are cognitively delayed. The individual must be able to conceptualize the indications of the PCA pump itself and its ability to relieve pain.

Prior to initiating a PCA pump for a patient, adequate analgesia must already have been provided. It is not practical to start the pump if a patient is already experiencing pain, especially moderate to severe in nature. Presurgical education is necessary when introducing PCA pumps within the surgical plan. Education must include not only the patient but also the family. Such education must include explicit directions that only the patient should push the PCA button to deliver the opioid analgesia regardless of the circumstances.

Overall, PCAs have been shown to be comparable, if not more effective, than conventional opioid administration. A meta-synthesis conducted by Hudcova, McNicol, Quah, Lau, and Carr (2006) discovered that patients who used PCA pumps experienced better pain control and satisfaction with their care, as opposed to those who received as-needed administration of opioids. Side effects were fairly similar between the groups, with the exception of increased incidence of pruritus in the PCA using patients. It is of note that there was a significantly higher use of

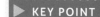

> ▶ **KEY POINT**

More than half of the individuals who misuse opioids have obtained the opioid through an individual (family member or friend) who was legally prescribed the opioid (Substance Abuse and Mental Health Services Administration, 2014). This alone demonstrates that providers are prescribing far too many opioids than what is necessary for the individual. Thus, the need for safe and effective prescribing policies and communication is necessary for those who will be administering opioid analgesia.

opioid analgesics among patients with a PCA pump. Therefore, careful monitoring of patients who use PCA pumps for postoperative analgesia is necessary to maintain safety in conjunction with adequate analgesic effect.

Peripheral Nerve Block and Local Anesthetics

Peripheral nerve blocks are widely used in postoperative pain management. A peripheral nerve block is the delivery of anesthetic agents to a specific peripheral nerve to block pain signaling in a defined region and can be administered as an intermittent injection or via a continuous pump. They are quite effective in managing regional pain, such as pain confined to a particular surgical area because the anesthetic is delivered directly to the injured nerve. The benefit of using a peripheral nerve block is to facilitate early ambulation and overall rehabilitation and recovery after a traumatic event, such as an extensive surgical procedure (McMahon, Koltzenburg, Tracey, & Turk, 2013). Peripheral nerve blocks are good alternatives for patients who are at an increased risk of respiratory depression secondary to opioid analgesia, those who want to avoid systemic medication administration, and those who are not responsive to oral routes of medication administration (Chang & White, 2017). In addition, peripheral nerve blocks can be used intraoperatively to decrease the amount of general anesthesia delivered, as well as opioid-sparing effects.

It is vital that the provider who is performing the peripheral nerve block be appropriately trained and experienced. Though peripheral nerve blocks have demonstrated to be effective, it is of note that they are still less widely performed because of increased time and expertise needed for placement (Jeon, 2012). Incorrect placement of the peripheral nerve block may lead to not only inadequately managed pain (10% to 15%) but also negative outcomes such as nerve injury (Liguori, 2004). Though peripheral nerve injury is relatively rare (<0.3%), it is important to discuss the risk with the patient prior to the procedure (Hardman, 2015). Other complications of peripheral nerve block include infection, catheter removal, hematoma, secondary injury from placement, and local anesthetic systemic toxicity (Chang & White, 2017; Jeng, Torrillo, & Rosenblatt, 2010).

Epidural Analgesia

Epidural analgesia is delivered via a catheter inserted into the epidural space. It is often used as a supplement to general anesthesia for surgical procedures or as the primary mode of anesthesia for surgeries involving the mediastinum to lower extremities and to provide analgesia in the hospital setting, including peripartum and palliative care. Proper care and assessment must be taken when an individual has an epidural catheter to reduce the risk of infection, leakage, and risk of dislodgement and subsequent pain. Frequent assessment of neurologic status, including sensation to temperature and touch, is necessary to provide adequate analgesia safely. Side effects include spinal headaches, pruritus, and hypotension, which may need intervention by fluid bolus. Despite its known efficacy, Hermandies, Hollmann, Stevens, and Lirk (2012) posit that failed anesthesia via epidural may be higher than previously thought, occurring in up to 30% of individuals. Reasons of failure may include incorrect placement, inadequate analgesia, and/or secondary migration of the catheter out of the epidural space. With correct placement, effective analgesia and blockade is dependent on the epidural solution, amount and concentration of the analgesic, local anesthetic, and/or adjuvant drug.

A three-medication "cocktail" for epidural administration, which aids in pain relief by working synergistically, may include a local anesthetic, an opioid, and adrenaline or clonidine. The most common example of this pharmaceutical combination is bupivacaine, fentanyl, and adrenaline (McMahon et al., 2013). The local anesthetic that is most often used in epidural infusions is bupivacaine. Its mechanism of action is to stabilize the neuronal membranes and prevent pain transmission and initiation of nerve impulses (Moore, Bridenbaugh, Bridenbaugh, & Tucker, 1970). Fentanyl, which is the most often used opioid in epidural infusion, works by acting upon the mu opioid receptors within the CNS, thereby suppressing pain transmission to the CNS (Micromedex Solutions, 2017b). Epinephrine is a strong vasopressor, which works on alpha- and beta-adrenergic receptors; it counters vasodilation and increased vascular permeability (Micromedex Solutions, 2017a).

Studies investigating the synergetic effect of the three-medication mixture demonstrate prolonged analgesic effects with no significant side effects, compared to use with these drugs alone (Becker & Reed, 2006; Connelly et al., 2011; Gurbet, Turker, Kose, & Uckunkaya, 2005; Prasad et al., 2016; Syal, Dogra, Ohri, Chauhan, & Goel, 2011). A study conducted by Gurbet et al. (2005) compared a control group of individual local anesthetics versus a combination group of anesthetic and opioid for women in labor. Those who received the bupivacaine and fentanyl via epidural had significantly prolonged spinal analgesia. In addition, low doses of fentanyl (12.5 µg) were optimal and sufficient to prolonging anesthetic effects.

With the addition of a vasopressor, such as adrenaline/epinephrine, the rate of absorption of local anesthetics is delayed and peak levels reduced (Becker & Reed, 2006). Early studies conducted by Moore, Liu, Pollock, Neal, and Knab (1998) concluded that the addition of epinephrine with bupivacaine prolongs the sensory block. Connelly et al. (2011) examined the effects of adding epinephrine to a bupivacaine epidural in early laboring women. It was determined that with the addition of epinephrine, there was a longer time to redose bupivacaine and decreased pain scores at 2.5 hours and 4.5 hours ($P < 0.04$), with no effect on labor outcomes and/or epinephrine side effects (Connelly et al., 2011). In general, mixing the bupivacaine with epidural increases the length of duration for the anesthetic itself and overall effective pain relief (Darshan et al., 2014). The addition of epinephrine in a peripheral nerve block or epidural slows absorption of local anesthetics and actively produces analgesia. It also aids in lowering the dose of local anesthetics and opioids administered, thus reducing the incidence of respiratory depression, sedation, nausea, vomiting, urinary retention, opioid-induced constipation, and orthostatic hypotension (McMahon et al., 2013).

The addition of clonidine in epidural infusions also provided benefits for women who were in labor. The benefits include dose-sparing effects of bupivacaine and prolonged duration of analgesia (Syal et al., 2011). As with other aforementioned studies, there were no negative side effects with the addition of clonidine. A recent study by Prasad et al. (2016) examined women undergoing gynecologic surgery. This study found that clonidine added to epidural anesthesia provided faster onset and prolonged sensory block duration, with no postoperative complications.

Nonopioid Analgesia

Considering the possibility of side effects and negative outcomes of opioid administration, nonopioids may be useful in managing postoperative pain. The use of nonopioids in addition to or in the absence of opioids is important and can have tremendous opioid-sparing effects. Common nonopioids used postoperatively may include nonsteroidal anti-inflammatory drugs (NSAIDs) and acetaminophen. These are useful considering they are over-the-counter drugs and the patient will be able to manage their pain postdischarge.

Nonsteroidal Anti-inflammatory Drugs

NSAIDs are effective at managing mild to moderate pain, through inhibition of peripheral and central cyclooxygenase (COX), but this does not come without side effects (McMahon et al., 2013). The enzyme COX-1 is often found in many tissues throughout the body and has several homeostatic functions, whereas COX-2 is generally induced and in high concentrations in the presence of inflammation. Inflammatory events induced by injury and surgical procedure usually involve proinflammatory mediators (i.e., cytokines, interleukins) and the production of nerve growth factors (Tal, 1999). COX, which is responsible for the production of prostanoids, thromboxane and prostaglandins, causes inflammation and subsequently associated pain. By inhibiting inflammation, pain is essentially relieved (Eisenach, Curry, Rauck, Pan, & Yaksh, 2010). It is important to note that NSAIDs, though effective, are nonselective and inhibit both COX-1 and COX-2, which makes adverse side effects, particularly gastrointestinal, more prevalent.

A common nonselective COX inhibitor used throughout the perioperative period is ketorolac. The use of ketorolac is opioid sparing and reduces opioid consumption by 25% to 45% (Garimella & Cellini, 2013). Because of its NSAID properties, this medication should not be used long term and may be contraindicated in certain surgical procedures postoperatively, owing to the increased bleeding risk (United States Food and Drug Administration, 2004). It is contraindicated as a prophylactic analgesia for this reason. The addition of a protective drug such as histamine 2 blockers and proton pump inhibitors with the use of COX inhibitors may be beneficial to ensure overall benefit and compliance with use (Portenoy, 2000).

Acetaminophen

Acetaminophen, though used often for mild to moderate pain, does not have anti-inflammatory properties or subsequent side effects, such as with NSAIDs. Therefore, acetaminophen does not have the same bleeding risks that are associated with NSAIDs. Though this is true, there are significant risks of hepatotoxicity.

Acetaminophen is metabolized in the liver and as such patients should not exceed 4 g of acetaminophen daily. Acetaminophen can be administered orally, rectally, or intravenously (paracetamol). Oral is generally the most common method of administration, but because of its slow onset of action, it may not be ideal in the acute postoperative period (Garimella & Cellini, 2013). Acetaminophen does possess opioid-sparing effects and works synergistically with other opioids. It is often paired with opioids in several combination formularies, such as Lortab and Norco, which combine hydrocodone and acetaminophen. When prescribing these combination medications, it is important that the patient receives the medication in intervals that will not exceed 4 g of acetaminophen per day in adults, or 75 mg/kg/d in children. Exceeding these maximum doses puts the patient at risk of developing hepatotoxicity.

Complementary Alternative Medicine

CAM therapy is unique, considering it is nonpharmacologic in nature. The use of CAM with an established treatment plan may enhance the effects of pharmacologic therapies. The following will discuss two frequently used CAMs for postoperative pain with documented efficacy: acupuncture and massage. Aside from these two commonly used CAMs, there are several others, including distraction, relaxation breathing, heat/cold application, aromatherapy, hypnosis, feedback, mindfulness, and exercise.

A staple in Eastern cultures, acupuncture is an ancient Chinese medical practice that may be beneficial in managing postoperative pain. Acupuncture is a relatively safe method when compared to opioid analgesia and may even have opioid-sparing effects. Though its side effects are minimal, it is important to note that practitioners of acupuncture must be specially trained to ensure safety. Associated side effects include nausea, vomiting, local skin irritation (bruising, swelling, bleeding, and/or pain at the injection site), needle breakage, and headaches. Although such side effects are more common, rare events include but are not limited to pneumothorax, spinal cord injury, hepatitis B, sepsis, and injury to internal organs (Chung, Bui, & Mills, 2003).

Though the biologic implications of acupuncture are not well understood, several studies have implicated acupuncture as being a useful therapy in the management of postoperative pain. An in-depth systemic review conducted by Sun, Gan, Dubose, and Habib (2008) examined the effects of acupuncture on postoperative pain and opioid-sparing effects. It was determined that individuals who received acupuncture postoperatively had significantly decreased opioid consumption and their pain intensity was decreased as well when compared to a control group. Subsequent opioid-related side effects were also significantly decreased. Further analysis and systematic review of the efficacy of acupuncture in postoperative pain management indicates that acupuncture is likely effective in managing pain and decreasing opioid consumption (Wu et al., 2016).

Massage therapy is one of the most often prescribed CAM approaches to pain management, most beneficial and least likely to be harmful to the patient (Adams,

White, & Beckett, 2010; Ezzo, 2007). Biopsychosocial factors, such as pain catastrophizing, anxiety, and high levels of stress, can impact a person's healing and lead to increased pain perception (Ezzo, 2007). Massage not only works as a stress relief, but also has biologic and physiologic properties to promote healing and analgesia, with minimal side effects. Most side effects that occur with nontraditional (non-Swedish) massage are often performed by incompetent and inexperienced therapists. These adverse effects include "cerebrovascular accidents, nerve damage, pulmonary embolism, and various pain syndromes" (McMahon et al., 2013). These adverse events rarely occur under the guidance of licensed massage therapist.

The primary effect of massage, which is relaxation, additionally may increase the efficacy of massage. The overall reduction of stress and psycho-physiologic arousal is beneficial for pain perception and healing (Ezzo, 2007; Richards, 1998). Massage has been used for many years with its biologic benefits known. Physiologic responses of relaxation include decreased blood pressure, lower oxygen demand, and decreased volumes of circulating cortisol and noradrenaline (Benson, 1975). Biologically, there is postulation that the gate-control theory of pain may be responsible for the mechanism of massage therapy. In essence, massage stimulates large diameter nerve fibers, which may inhibit transmission of noxious stimuli and diminish pain perception (Ezzo, 2007). Massage has the ability to garner increased blood flow locally and reduce muscle tone and tension (McMahon et al., 2013). In addition, massage may have anti-inflammatory benefits, which may provide relief in muscular injuries. After muscular damage, an inflammatory response ensues with the release of macrophages and other proinflammatory cell mediators. A study conducted by Waters et al. (2011) demonstrated that the magnitude of applied load affects resident (M2) and nonresident (M1) macrophage numbers within the muscle, thus suggesting an improved healing and regenerating environment with massage. Furthermore, massage may be effective in reducing cellular infiltration and the resulting inflammation and edema, which may lead to increased pain perception (Butterfield, Best, & Merrick, 2006).

▌Adjuvants and PPP

Adjuvants are defined as medications that may work synergistically with opioid and nonopioid analgesics. Examples of adjuvants include antidepressants, anticonvulsants, and cannabinoids for pain management. Although these medications are not used in the immediate postoperative period, they are commonly prescribed for patients with persistent neuropathic pain.

▌Antidepressants

There is a correlation between chronic pain and depression, which has been demonstrated in various studies. Those who suffer from chronic pain in general are 5 times more likely to suffer from depression than healthy controls (Gureje, Von Korff, Simon, & Gater, 1998). Considering the increased incidence of depression in chronic pain sufferers, it is difficult for clinicians to determine whether depression is a result of chronic pain, vice versa, or completely independent of each other. Because of the connectedness of depression and chronic pain, the novelty of using antidepressants to manage pain is feasible. In fact, much of what researchers know about antidepressants and their influence on pain is based upon their treatment of psychiatric disorders such as depression (McMahon et al., 2013). One must also be aware that the relationship is not exclusive considering that most tricyclic antidepressants, which are used to treat pain, are done so at a much lower dose than those used to treat depression. Furthermore, depression is not always present in those who experience pain relief through the use of antidepressant therapies (McMahon et al., 2013; Sansone & Sansone, 2008).

Anticonvulsants

Chronic pain, particularly pain from neuropathic pain states, is categorized by ectopic firing of neuronal impulses. Epilepsy and other seizure disorders are characterized by a similar mechanism. This CNS disorder is characterized by erroneous firing of cortical neurons, resulting in seizures varying in degree (i.e., focal, grand mal). Essentially, neuroplasticity is affected in both seizure disorders and chronic pain (Wiffen et al., 2005). There are many similarities between the pathophysiologic phenomena in epilepsy models and neuropathic pain models, which justify the use of anticonvulsant therapy in the maintenance of chronic pain (Tremont-Lukats, Megeff, & Backonja, 2000; Wiffen et al., 2005).

Cannabinoids

Cannabinoids may be preferred over some analgesics, or adjunctively, particularly with opioids because of their high risk of associated side effects. Opioids have an increased risk of sedation, loss of appetite, nausea, OIH, constipation, respiratory depression, as well as issues with tolerance and dependence. Cannabinoids may negate these side effects (Elikottil, Gupta, & Gupta, 2009). Cannabinoids do not have these specific side effects; rather, they act as both an antiemetic and appetite stimulant within the clinical setting. Cannabinoids, specifically Sativex, are also helpful in improving not only pain, but mood, daily functioning, and sleep (Nurmikko et al., 2007). This is not to say that they do not come without their own associated side effects. Immediate side effects are dizziness and mood alterations, and research has shown prolonged use may precede psychosis and/or schizophrenia, particularly in those who begin marijuana ingestion at an early age (McMahon et al., 2013; Schneider, 2008). There is also a potential risk of misuse and addiction in habitual cannabis users.

Special Considerations

Cultural Considerations

▶ Perception and expression of pain differ among various racial and ethnic groups, based on differences in expectations and acceptance of pain (Peacock & Patel, 2008).

▶ Experimental pain is greater in Black Americans than non-Hispanic White Americans, though translatability is in question (Kim et al., 2017).

Table 10-4. Patient/Family Education Points Regarding Opioids

Take medications as prescribed and do not share prescribed medications.

Monitor for side effects of analgesic medications. Call 911 if any serious side effects, such as respiratory depression and/or loss of consciousness.

Dispose of all opioid medications appropriately.
- There are local, secure drop-offs of medications scheduled within local communities.
- If unable to do this, remove identifiable information, dissolve pills within the original container (may need to crush), and fill container with undesirable substance, such as cat litter or sand. Then put this container in a nonidentifiable container (such as a yogurt carton) and dispose.
- Do *not* flush medications.

National Guidelines for Managing Postoperative Pain (Position Statement)

▶ Management of Postoperative Pain: A Clinical Practice Guideline from the American Pain Society, the American Society of Regional Anesthesia and Pain Medicine, and the American Society of Anesthesiologists' Committee on Regional Anesthesia, Executive Committee, and Administrative Council (Chou et al., 2016).

Patient/Family Education

Table 10-4 outlines the education points for the patient and family.

▶ **KEY POINTS**

- When prescribing opioids, ensure that family adheres to plan and monitors for signs and symptoms of addiction, tolerance, and/or withdrawal.
- Set realistic pain goals with the patient and family and include within this education, a taper plan particularly when prescribing opioids.
- Anticipate painful activities and/or procedures and premedicate if necessary.
- Discuss the importance of follow-up care to ensure proper healing and resolution of pain beyond the acute period.

REFERENCES

Adams, R., White, B., & Beckett, C. (2010). The effects of massage therapy on pain management in the acute care setting. *International Journal of Therapeutic Massage & Bodywork, 3*(1), 4–11.

Becker, D. E., & Reed, K. L. (2006). Essentials of local anesthetic pharmacology. *Anesthesia Progress, 53*(3), 98–108; quiz 109–110. doi:10.2344/0003-3006(2006)53[98:Eolap]2.0.Co;2

Benson, H. (1975). *The relaxation response.* New York, NY: William Morrow & Company.

Bottemiller, S. (2012). Opioid-induced hyperalgesia: An emerging treatment challenge. *U.S. Pharmacist, 37*(5), HS2–HS7.

Brennan, F., Carr, D. B., & Cousins, M. (2007). Pain management: A fundamental human right. *Anesthesia & Analgesia, 105*(1), 205–221. doi:10.1213/01.ane.0000268145.52345.55

Butterfield, T. A., Best, T. M., & Merrick, M. A. (2006). The dual roles of neutrophils and macrophages in inflammation: A critical balance between tissue damage and repair. *Journal of Athletic Training, 41*(4), 457–465.

Chakravorty, S., & Williams, T. N. (2015). Sickle cell disease: A neglected chronic disease of increasing global health importance. *Archives of Disease in Childhood, 100*(1), 48–53.

Chang, A., White, B. A. (2017). *Peripheral nerve blocks.* [Updated 2017 Oct 6]. StatPearls [Internet]. Treasure Island, FL: StatPearls. Retrieved from https://www.ncbi.nlm.nih.gov/books/NBK459210/

Chou, R., Gordon, D. B., de Leon-Casasola, O. A., Rosenberg, J. M., Bickler, S., Brennan, T., . . . Wu, C. L. (2016). Management of postoperative pain: A clinical practice guideline from the American Pain Society, the American Society of Regional Anesthesia and Pain Medicine, and the American Society of Anesthesiologists' Committee on Regional Anesthesia, Executive Committee, and Administrative Council. *The Journal of Pain, 17*(2), 131–157. doi:10.1016/j.jpain.2015.12.008

Chung, A., Bui, L., & Mills, E. (2003). Adverse effects of acupuncture. Which are clinically significant? *Canadian Family Physician, 49*, 985–989.

Connelly, N. R., Freiman, J. P., Lucas, T., Parker, R. K., Raghunathan, K., Gibson, C., . . . Iwashita, C. (2011). Addition of epinephrine to epidural bupivacaine infusions following initiation of labor analgesia with epidural fentanyl. *Journal of Clinical Anesthesia, 23*(4), 265–269. doi:10.1016/j.jclinane.2010.09.005

Darshan, M., Sri Devi, S., Karthik, A., Jeyakumar, V., Karthik, M., & Nagasunitha, C. (2014). Epinephrine as epidural adjuvant to bupivacaine and fentanyl in elective orthopedic surgeries. *Scholars Journal of Applied Medical Sciences, 2*(2), 1540–1550.

Eisenach, M. D. J. C., Curry, R. N. R., Rauck, M. D. R., Pan, M. D. P., & Yaksh, P. D. T. L. (2010). Role of spinal cyclooxygenase in human postoperaive and chronic pain. *Anesthesiology, 112*(5), 1225–1233. doi:10.1097/ALN.0b013e3181d94dc0

Elikottil, J., Gupta, P., & Gupta, K. (2009). The analgesic potential of cannabinoids. *Journal of Opioid Management, 5*(6), 341–357.

Ezzo, J. (2007). What can be learned from Cochrane systematic reviews of massage that can guide future research? *Journal of Alternative and Complementary Medicine, 13*(2), 291–295. doi:10.1089/act.2007.13604

Feldman, C. H., Dong, Y., Katz, J. N., Donnell-Fink, L. A., & Losina, E. (2015). Association between socioeconomic status and pain function and pain catastrophizing at presentation for total knee arthroplasty. *BMC Musculoskeletal Disorders, 16*, 18.

Fillingim, R. B., King, C. D., Ribeiro-Dasilva, M. C., Rahim-Williams, B., & Riley, J. L., 3rd. (2009). Sex, gender, and pain: A review of recent clinical and experimental findings. *Pain, 10*(5), 447–485.

Garimella, V., & Cellini, C. (2013). Postoperative pain control. *Clinics in Colon and Rectal Surgery, 26*(3), 191–196. doi:10.1055/s-0033-1351138

Gatchel, R. J., Peng, Y. B., Peters, M. L., Fuchs, P. N., & Turk, D. C. (2007). The biopsychosocial approach to chronic pain: Scientific advances and future directions. *Psychological Bulletin, 133*(4), 581–624.

Gerbershagen, H. J., Pogatzki-Zahn, E., Aduckathil, S., Peelen, L. M., Kappen, T. H., van Wijck, A. J. M., . . . Meissner, W. (2014). Procedure-specific risk factor analysis for the development of severe postoperative pain. *Anesthesiology, 120*(5), 1237–1245. doi:10.1097/ALN.0000000000000108

Gupta, A., Kaur, K., Sharma, S., Goyal, S., Arora, S., & Murthy, R. S. R. (2010). Clinical aspects of acute post-operative pain management and its assessment. *Journal of Advanced Pharmaceutical Technology & Research, 1*(2), 97–108.

Gurbet, A., Turker, G., Kose, D. O., & Uckunkaya, N. (2005). Intrathecal epinephrine in combined spinal-epidural analgesia for labor: Dose-response relationship for epinephrine added to a local anesthetic-opioid combination. *International Journal of Obstetric Anesthesia, 14*(2), 121–125. doi:10.1016/j.ijoa.2004.12.002

Gureje, O., Von Korff, M., Simon, G. E., & Gater, R. (1998). Persistent pain and well-being: A World Health Organization Study in Primary Care. *JAMA, 280*(2), 147–151.

Hardman, D. (2015). Nerve injury after peripheral nerve block: Best practices and medical-legal protection strategies. *Anesthesiology News, 7*(1), 1–7.

Hermandies, J., Hollmann, M. W., Stevens, M. F., & Lirk, P. (2012). Failed epidural: Causes and management. *British Journal of Anaesthesia, 109*(2), 144–154.

Hudcova, J., McNicol, E., Quah, C., Lau, J., & Carr, D. B. (2006). Patient controlled opioid analgesia versus conventional opioid analgesia for postoperative pain. *Cochrane Database of Systematic Reviews* (4), CD003348. doi:10.1002/14651858.CD003348.pub2

International Association for the Study of Pain. (1994). Classification of chronic pain. Descriptions of chronic pain syndromes and definitions of pain terms. *Pain, 3*(S1), S1–S226.

Jeng, C. L., Torrillo, T. M., & Rosenblatt, M. A. (2010). Complications of peripheral nerve blocks. *British Journal of Anaesthesia, 105*(S1), i97–i107.

Jeon, Y.-T. (2012). Peripheral nerve block for anesthesia in patients having knee arthroplasty. *Korean Journal of Anesthesiology, 62*(5), 403–404. doi:10.4097/kjae.2012.62.5.403

Kehlet, H., Jensen, T. S., & Woolf, C. J. (2006). Persistent postsurgical pain: Risk factors and prevention. *Lancet, 367*(9522), 1618–1625. doi:10.1016/s0140-6736(06)68700-x

Kim, H. J., Yang, G. S., Greenspan, J. D., Downton, K. D., Griffith, K. A., Renn, C. L., . . . Dorsey, S. G. (2017). Racial and ethnic differences in experimental pain sensitivity: Systematic review and meta-analysis. *Pain, 158*(2), 194–211. doi:10.1097/j .pain.0000000000000731

Liguori, G. A. (2004). Complications of regional anesthesia: Nerve injury and peripheral neural blockade. *Journal of Neurosurgical Anesthesiology, 16*(1), 84–86.

Logan, D. E., & Rose, J. (2005). Is postoperative pain a self-fulfilling prophecy? Expectancy effects on postoperative pain and patient-controlled analgesia use among adolescent surgical patients. *Journal of Pediatric Psychology, 30*(2), 187–196.

Macrae, W. A. (2001). Chronic pain after surgery. *BJA: International Journal of Anaesthesia, 87*(1), 88–98.

McMahon, S. B., Koltzenburg, M., Tracey, I., & Turk, D. (2013). *Wall & Melzack's textbook of pain* (6th ed.). Philadelphia, PA: Elsevier.

Merkel, S. I., Voepel-Lewis, T., Shayevitz, J. R., & Malviya, S. (1997). The FLACC: A behavioral scale for scoring postoperative pain in young children. *Pediatric Nursing, 23*(3), 293–297.

Micromedex Solutions. (2017a). *Epinephrine.* Ann Arbor, MI: Truven Health Analytics. Retrieved from http://www.micromedexsolutions.com

Micromedex Solutions. (2017b). *Fentanyl.* Ann Arbor, MI: Truven Health Analytics. Retrieved from http://www.micromedexsolutions.com.

Moore, D. C., Bridenbaugh, L., Bridenbaugh, P. O., & Tucker, G. T. (1970). Bupivacaine: A review of 2,077 cases. *JAMA, 214*(4), 713–718. doi:10.1001/jama.1970.03180040021003

Moore, J. M., Liu, S. S., Pollock, J. E., Neal, J. M., & Knab, J. H. (1998). Epinephrine prolongs bupivacaine spinal anesthesia. *Anesthesia and Analgesia, 86*(2S), 295S. doi:10.1097/00000539-199802001-00293

Niraj, G., & Rowbotham, D. J. (2011). Persistent postoperative pain: Where are we now? *British Journal of Anaesthesia, 107*(1), 25–29. doi:10.1093/bja/aer116

Nurmikko, T. J., Serpell, M. G., Hoggart, B., Toomey, P. J., Morlion, B. J., & Haines, D. (2007). Sativex successfully treats neuropathic pain characterised by allodynia: A randomised, double-blind, placebo-controlled clinical trial. *Pain, 133*(1–3), 210–220. doi:10.1016/j. pain.2007.08.028

Pasero, C. (2009). Assessment of sedation during opioid administration for pain management. *Journal of PeriAnesthesia Nursing, 24*(3), 186–190.

Pathan, H., & Williams, J. (2012). Basic opioid pharmacology: An update. *British Journal of Pain, 6*(1), 11–16. doi:10.1177/2049463712438493

Peacock, S., & Patel, S. (2008). Cultural influences on pain. *Reviews in Pain, 1*(2), 6–9. doi:10.1177/204946370800100203

Perry, M., Starkweather, A., Baumbauer, K., & Young, E. (2018). Factors leading to persistent postsurgical pain in adolescents undergoing spinal fusion: An integrative literature review. *Journal of Pediatric Nursing, 38*, 74–80. doi:10.1016/j.pedn.2017.10.013

Phillips, D. M. (2000). JCAHO pain management standards are unveiled. Joint Commission on Accreditation of Healthcare Organizations. *JAMA, 284*(4), 428–429.

Portenoy, R. K. (2000). Current pharmacotherapy of chronic pain. *Journal of Pain Symptom Management, 19*(1 Suppl.), S16–S20.

Prasad, R., Rao, R., Turai, A., Prabha, P., Shreyavathi, R., & Harsoor, K. (2016). Effect of epidural clonidine on characteristics of spinal anaesthesia in patients undergoing gynaecological surgeries: A clinical study. *Indian Journal of Anaesthesia, 60*(6), 398–402. doi:10.4103/0019-5049.183395

Rabbitts, J. A., Fisher, E., Rosenbloom, B. N., & Palermo, T. M. (2017). Prevalence and predictors of chronic postsurgical pain in children: A systematic review and meta-analysis. *Journal of Pain, 18*(6), 605–614. doi:10.1016/j.jpain.2017.03.007

Richards, K. C. (1998). Effect of a back massage and relaxation intervention on sleep in critically ill patients. *American Journal of Critical Care, 7*(4), 288–299.

Sansone, R. A., & Sansone, L. A. (2008). Pain, pain, go away: Antidepressants and pain management. *Psychiatry (Edgmont), 5*(12), 16–19.

Schneider, M. (2008). Puberty as a highly vulnerable developmental period for the consequences of cannabis exposure. *Addiction Biology, 13*(2), 253–263. doi:10.1111/j.1369-1600.2008.00110.x

Substance Abuse and Mental Health Services Administration. (2014). *Alcohol, tobacco, and other drugs.* Retrieved from https://www.samhsa.gov/atod/opioids

Sun, Y., Gan, T. J., Dubose, J. W., & Habib, A. S. (2008). Acupuncture and related techniques for postoperative pain: A systematic review of randomized controlled trials. *British Journal of Anaesthesia, 101*(2), 151–160. doi:10.1093/bja/aen146

Syal, K., Dogra, R. K., Ohri, A., Chauhan, G., & Goel, A. (2011). Epidural labour analgesia using Bupivacaine and Clonidine. *Journal of Anaesthesiology, Clinical Pharmacology, 27*(1), 87–90.

Tal, M. (1999). A role for inflammation in chronic pain. *Current Review of Pain, 3*(6), 440–446.

Tremont-Lukats, I. W., Megeff, C., & Backonja, M. M. (2000). Anticonvulsants for neuropathic pain syndromes: Mechanisms of action and place in therapy. *Drugs, 60*(5), 1029–1052.

United States Department of Health and Human Services. (2017). *What is the US opioid epidemic?* Retrieved from https://www.hhs.gov/opioids/about-the-epidemic/index.html

United States Food and Drug Administration. (2004). *Vioxx (rofecoxib) questions and answers.* Retrieved from https://www.fda.gov/drugs/drugsafety/postmarketdrugsafetyinformation-forpatientsandproviders/ucm106290.htm

Ventafridda, V., Saita, L., Ripamonti, C., & De Conno, F. (1985). WHO guidelines for the use of analgesics in cancer pain. *International Journal of Tissue Reactions, 7*(1), 93–96.

Wandner, L., Scipio, C. D., Hirsch, A. T., Morais, C. A., & Robinson, M. E. (2012). The perception of pain in others: How gender, race and age influence pain expectations. *Journal of Pain, 13*(3), 220–227.

Wiffen, P. J., Derry, S., Moore, R. A., Aldington, D., Cole, P., Rice, A. S., . . . Kalso, E. A. (2013). Antiepileptic drugs for neuropathic pain and fibromyalgia—An overview of Cochrane reviews. *Cochrane Database of Systematic Review,* (11), CD010567. doi:10.1002/14651858 .CD010567.pub2

Wiffen, P., Collins, S., McQuay, H., Carroll, D., Jadad, A., & Moore, A. (2005). Anticonvulsant drugs for acute and chronic pain. *Cochrane Database of Systematic Review*, (3), CD001133. doi:10.1002/14651858.CD001133.pub2

Williams, G., Howard, R. F., & Liossi, C. (2017). Persistent postsurgical pain in children and young people: Prediction, prevention, and management. *Pain Reports, 2*(5), e616. doi:10.1097/PR9.0000000000000616

Wong-Baker Faces Foundation. (2016). *Wong-Baker FACES® pain rating scale.* Retrieved from http://www.WongBakerFACES.org

World Health Organization. (1986). *Cancer pain relief.* Geneva: Author.

Wu, M.-S., Chen, K.-H., Chen, I. F., Huang, S. K., Tzeng, P.-C., Yeh, M.-L., . . . Chen, C. (2016). The efficacy of acupuncture in post-operative pain management: A systematic review and meta-analysis. *PLoS One, 11*(3), e0150367. doi:10.1371/journal.pone.0150367

CHAPTER 11

TREATING PAIN IN THE PATIENT WITH CURRENT OR PAST HISTORY OF DEPENDENCE SYNDROME

Thomas M. Julian

Introduction

Pain management is a complex and challenging aspect of nursing care and in the case of individuals who are experiencing comorbid pain and substance use disorders (SUDs), the difficulties and complexities are much greater. The field of pain management has been continuously evolving over the past three decades, with the most significant trends in pain medicine comprising an increasing emphasis on aggressive treatment of acute and chronic pain with prescription opiate/opioid medications beginning in the mid-1990s and the subsequent opiate use epidemic that has evolved into the greatest public health crisis of the 21st century. The great emphasis placed on treating pain as the "fifth vital sign" that arose in the medical field in the late 1990s found support in JCAHO practice regulations (2001) that held hospitals accountable for pain control as a patient outcome. These trends in the pain management field were accompanied by a significant increase in opioid prescriptions, beginning with the marketing of oxycontin in 1996, and increasing steadily in the early 2000s (Centers for Disease Control and Prevention [CDC], 2011). The general consensus within the field of pain research saw prescription opioids as the "gold standard" treatment, first-line interventions for acute postsurgical pain as well as chronic cancer-related pain syndromes. During this time period, these painkillers were increasingly being employed as first-line pharmacologic treatment interventions for a myriad of chronic pain syndromes. Although the safety and efficacy of opioids in acute postsurgical and cancer pain were supported by a strong body of research, evidence for the safety and efficacy of opioid painkillers in the treatment of chronic noncancer pain was much more tenuous; this did not stop them from being widely marketed and prescribed to treat chronic pain. At this point, recognition of the increasing prevalence of addiction to prescription opiate/opioid painkillers that followed the increase in opioid prescriptions for chronic pain led some researchers and clinicians to begin to question the purported efficacy and safety of long-term opioid therapy for chronic pain patients. A landmark investigation by the Centers for Disease Control and Prevention (CDC), released in 2011, demonstrated that there was a strong association between the increasing rates of opioid overdose mortality and prescription painkiller-related emergency department admissions, and the corresponding increase in opioid prescriptions between 1999 and 2008 (Figure 11-1). At this time, prescription drug overdoses had surpassed illicit (heroin and cocaine) drug overdoses as the primary cause of drug overdose death, which was then second only to motor vehicle accidents as the primary cause of accidental death in the United States (CDC, 2011). The intervening years have seen an increasing recognition within the pain treatment field of the dangerous addictive potential of prescription painkillers, and the accompanying changes in the availability of prescription opioids for misuse has seen a significant trend of individuals with established opioid use disorders transitioning to misusing heroin (which is cheaper and more readily available), with resulting increases in heroin overdose deaths. The adulteration of the street heroin supply with the powerful synthetic opioid fentanyl (25-40 times more potent than

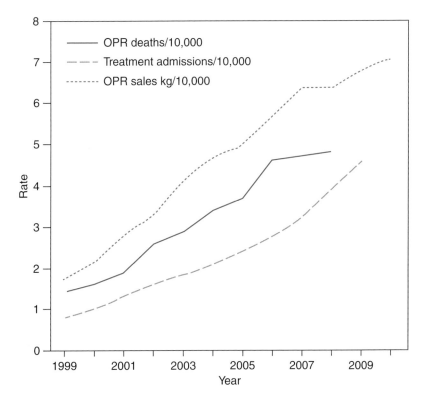

Figure 11–1. Rates of opioid pain reliever (OPR) overdose deaths, OPR treatment admissions and kilograms of OPR sold—United States 1999 to 2010. Rate implies age-adjusted rates per 100 000 population for OPR deaths, crude rates per 10 000 population for OPR abuse treatment admissions, and crude rates per 10 000 population for kilograms of OPR sold. Adapted from Centers for Disease Control and Prevention. (2011). Vital signs: Overdoses of prescription opioid pain relievers—United States, 1999–2008. *Morbidity and Mortality Weekly Report, 60*(43), 1487–1492.

heroin) has greatly increased opioid overdose mortality rates in the past few years so that drug overdose deaths (72 306 in 2017) have surpassed automobile accidents as the primary cause of accidental death in the country (National Center for Health Statistics, 2018). Opiate/opioids are involved in the majority of drug overdose deaths (49 068 in 2017), with the majority involving fentanyl-related fatalities (29 406 in 2017) (Figure 11-2). However, the ongoing contribution of prescription painkiller misuse to the opiate epidemic must not be underestimated as nearly 80% of Americans misusing heroin reported that they began their addiction using prescription painkillers (National Institute on Drug Abuse, National Institutes of Health, & U.S. Department of Health and Human Services, 2018).

█ Background

SUDs, also referred to as addiction disease, are a class of neurobiologic syndromes that are characterized by continued compulsive use of a drug (such as alcohol, cocaine, or prescription opiate painkillers), despite negative consequences to health, psychological well-being, and social functioning. Many legal (alcohol, tobacco) and illegal (marijuana, heroin, cocaine) drugs have the capacity to produce a pleasurable state of intoxication that is highly reinforcing of continued drug use. The psychologically rewarding effects of certain drugs have led to their recreational use by diverse cultures throughout human history. A certain percentage of individuals who engage in recreational drug use will progress to active addiction, where drug use becomes compulsive and involuntary and drug taking is increasingly motivated by relief of dysphoria rather than for pleasurable or euphoric effects. The demographics

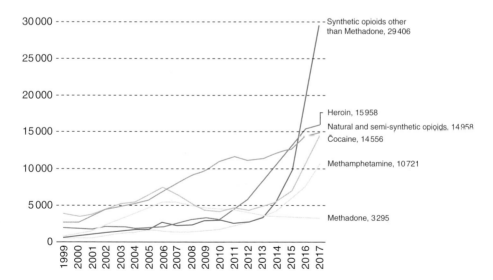

Figure 11–2. Drugs involved in U.S. overdose deaths, 1999 to 2017. Adapted from National Center for Health Statistics. (2018). *Overdose death rates 1999–2017*. Retrieved from https://www .drugabuse.gov/related-topics/trends-statistics/overdose-death-rates

of addiction disease in recent years have demonstrated an alarming increase in the prevalence of misuse of prescription and illicit opiate narcotics that have reached epidemic proportions and comprise a key public health emergency of great relevance to the field of pain management in the United States and other western societies (Volkow, Benveniste, & McLellan, 2018).

Addiction disease, including opiate use disorders (OUDs), affects a large segment of the population. Knowledge about the biology, epidemiology, and treatment modalities for addiction disease is therefore vital for the advanced practice nurse, especially within the context of management of acute and chronic pain patients. The 2017 National Survey on Drug Use and Health (NSUDH) commissioned by the Substance Abuse and Mental Health Services Administration (SAMSHA) contains the most current population level data on the disease burden of addiction and psychiatric disease in the American population. According to the NSUDH, in 2017, approximately 30.5 million Americans engaged in illicit drug use during the previous month (11.2% of the adult population over the age of 12). For young adults aged 18 to 25, the rate was much higher (25%). Past year illicit opioid use, defined as any use of illicit opiates (heroin), or use of prescription opiate or opioid narcotics without a prescription or in larger amounts or longer time than prescribed, was reported for 11.4 million Americans, comprising 4.2% of all adults and 7.3% of all young adults in the U.S. population (Substance Abuse and Mental Health Services Administration [SAMSHA], 2018) (Figure 11-3). The incidence of new opioid misusers was also alarming, as 2 million individuals initiated prescription painkiller misuse and 81 000 initiated heroin use during the past year. In 2017, 19.7 million (7.2%) adults met the criteria for a diagnosis of an SUD; of these, 7.5 million met criteria for an SUD for illicit drugs (SAMSHA, 2018). Although the rates of misuse of alcohol and most

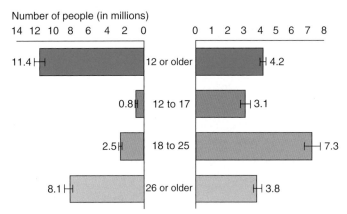

Figure 11-3. Past year opioid misuse among people aged 12 or older, by age group: 2017. Note: Opioid misuse is defined as heroin use or prescription pain reliever misuse. Adapted from Substance Abuse and Mental Health Services Administration. (2018). *Key substance use and mental health indicators in the United States: Results from the 2017 National Survey on Drug Use and Health* (HHS Publication No. SMA 18-5068, NSDUH Series H-53). Rockville, MD: Center for Behavioral Health Statistics and Quality, Substance Abuse and Mental Health Services Administration. Retrieved from https://www.samhsa.gov/data

illicit drugs (with the exception of marijuana) have remained stable over the past two decades, there has been an epidemic increase in the rates of misuse of prescription and illicit opiate/opioid narcotics. Approximately 2.1 million adults met the criterion for an OUD in 2017, with 1.7 million having a prescription drug SUD and 700 000 having a heroin use disorder; the rate of OUDs in the young adult population is now 1.3% (SAMSHA, 2018). Of the 6 million Americans (2.2% of the adult population) engaging in past month prescription drug misuse, the majority (3.2 million or 1.2% of adults) misused painkillers (opiate/opioid drugs), whereas 1.7 million misused tranquilizers (benzodiazepines), 1.8 million misused stimulants, and approximately 350 000 misused sedative drugs (SAMSHA, 2018) (Figure 11-4). The misuse of benzodiazepines is a phenomenon of particular importance to pain clinicians, as benzodiazepine overdose deaths increased 8-fold between 2002 and 2016 and the majority of these deaths also involved opioids (National Center for Health Statistics, 2018). The phenomenon of coaddiction to opioids and benzodiazepines or other sedative drugs should be of great concern to nurses working in pain management and addiction, as these combinations greatly increase a person's risk for a fatal drug overdose because of the synergistic effect on depression of the respiratory control centers in the central nervous system.

The high rate of SUDs is exacerbated by the insufficient treatment infrastructure for managing SUDs and comorbid psychiatric illnesses; of the 20.7 million Americans requiring treatment for SUDs in 2017, only 4 million (12.2%) received treatment. Even more alarming, of the 8.1 million Americans with an SUD and a comorbid psychiatric illness, only 8.3% received treatment for addiction and the comorbid mental illness and 49% received no treatment at all (SAMSHA, 2018). These data are concerning because an overwhelming body of research has demonstrated that addiction is a chronic, relapsing, degenerative neurobiologic disease that requires

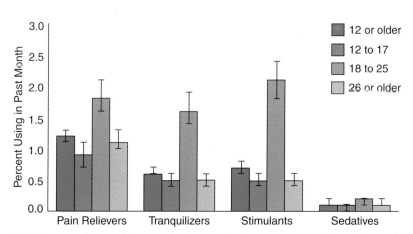

Figure 11–4. Past month prescription psychotherapeutic misuse among people aged 12 or older, by age group: Percentages, 2017. Adapted from Substance Abuse and Mental Health Services Administration. (2018). *Key substance use and mental health indicators in the United States: Results from the 2017 National Survey on Drug Use and Health* (HHS Publication No. SMA 18-5068, NSDUH Series H-53). Rockville, MD: Center for Behavioral Health Statistics and Quality, Substance Abuse and Mental Health Services Administration. Retrieved from https://www.samhsa.gov/data

ongoing treatment to preserve health and functional status and prevent relapse and death. The epidemiologic evidence has demonstrated that addiction disease is a common syndrome within the U.S. population and has shown that there is a high degree of overlap and comorbidity for addiction with chronic pain syndromes and many common psychiatric diseases (mood disorders, schizophrenia, attention deficit disorders). The presence of addiction disease within a patient being treated for a pain syndrome greatly complicates treatment for several reasons. The most obvious of these factors involves the addictive nature of the opiate/opioid analgesics that have traditionally been the primary pharmacologic treatment for both acute and chronic pain management. Careful attention in assessing and monitoring patients receiving pharmacologic treatments for pain management is a critical practice competency for nurse practitioners and advanced practice nurses. Patient assessment and risk stratification have been greatly assisted in recent years by the development of several screening instruments to measure addiction risk with opioid treatment. These instruments are summarized in the next section.

Patient Assessment and Screening Tools for Long-Term Opiate Treatment

This section of the chapter will describe the different screening instruments that have been developed to aid clinicians in making decisions related to the utilization of opiate/opioid analgesics in the context of pain management. The Pain Medication Questionnaire (PMQ) is a brief 26-item (Likert scale) self-report screening instrument designed to assess the risk of opioid medication misuse in chronic pain patients. Patients respond to each question on a 5-point Likert scale from 0 (disagree) to 4 (agree). The PMQ is designed to measure chronic pain patients on a range of potential risk based on endorsement of behaviors and attitudes correlated with opioid misuse, which were identified through addiction literature and expert consensus (Holmes et al., 2006). Scores on the PMQ range from 0 to 104, with increasing scores associated with greater risk of medication misuse. The PMQ was validated in a sample ($n = 271$) of new chronic pain patients. Patients are stratified by risk according to their total scale score, with a score between 70 and 104 indicating "high risk" and a score of 0 to 34 indicating "low risk." The original study showed that individuals in the "high risk PMQ" group were 2.6 times more likely to have a known substance use problem and 2.3 times more likely to drop out of treatment relative to individuals scoring in the "low risk PMQ" group (Holmes et al., 2006). Patients who completed the treatment period measured at 6 months after treatment completion were found to have significant decreases in their scores relative to patients who were unsuccessfully discharged from the pain management program or voluntarily dropped out (Holmes et al., 2006).

> ▶ **KEY POINT**
>
> Opioid therapy carries a risk of addiction that must be assessed by clinicians prior to initiation and regularly during follow-up.

The Risk Index for Overdose or Serious Opioid-Induced Respiratory Depression (RIOSORD) is a brief inventory that is intended as a screening tool to estimate the likelihood of life-threatening respiratory depression or overdose among medical users of prescription opioid painkillers. The RIOSORD was derived from a case–control analysis of healthcare data for 1 877 841 patients with an opioid prescription seen through the Veteran's Health Administration from October 2010 to September 2012, which identified 817 cases of overdose or severe respiratory depression and used regression modeling to compare predictor risk variables with 8170 controls. Point values were assigned to each predictor variable and modeling of risk index scores was performed to calculate predicted probabilities of OSORD (Zedler et al., 2015). The analyses identified 15 predictor variables which correlated with increased risk of respiratory depression, which were retained in the final version of the RIOSORD. Each predictor was assigned a specific point value (with the total scale score ranging from 0 to 110), with increasing scores indicating greater risk of overdose or respiratory depression. Ten risk classes by deciles of predicted probability were identified. Average predicted probabilities for adverse events ranged from 3% for the first decile (scores 0-24) to 94% for the 10th decile (scores $\geq$67) and these predicted probabilities were very similar to the observed incidence rates of 3% through 86% across risk classes (model C-statistic = 0.88) (Hosmer–Lemeshow goodness-of-fit statistic = 10.8, $P > 0.05$). The RIOSORD is intended for use as a screening tool to assess patient's baseline risk of opioid overdose or respiratory depression and can also be used at intervals during ongoing long-term opioid treatment and to reevaluate risk based on changes to patient clinical status or medication regimen.

The Current Opioid Misuse Measure (COMM) was created as a measure to assess chronic pain patients already receiving long-term opioid therapy for changes in health status over time (Butler et al., 2007). The COMM operationalizes changes in patient status through measurement of observable behaviors during a 30-day time period. The initial validation of the COMM scale was conducted in a sample ($n = 227$) receiving opioids for chronic noncancer pain. A 17-item version of the scale demonstrated adequate ability to measure aberrant drug-related behaviors and good internal consistency ($\alpha = 0.86$) and test–retest reliability (ICC = 0.86; 95% CI: 0.77-0.92), and was retained. With a total scale score range of 0 to 68, a cutoff score of 9 yielded a sensitivity of 0.77 and specificity of 0.66 (Butler et al., 2007). A cross validation of the COMM scale in a sample ($n = 226$) of chronic noncancer pain patients produced comparable results ($\alpha = 0.83$) (AUC = 0.79; SE = 0.31, 95% CI: 0.73-0.85, $P = 0.001$) (Butler, Budman, Fanciullo, & Jamison, 2010).

The Opioid Risk Tool (ORT) was created as a brief screening tool to predict aberrant drug-related behavior in chronic pain patients on long-term opioid therapy. The ORT measures risk factors, which were derived from the addiction research literature (personal/family history of SUDs, age, childhood sexual abuse history, and psychiatric diagnoses). Initial validation of the ORT was conducted in a sample ($n = 185$) of new pain clinic patients who received scores of 0 to 3 (low risk), 4 to 7 (moderate risk), or $\geq$8 (high risk) (Webster & Webster, 2005). The C-statistic (a measure of the sensitivity and specificity of the ORT screen) demonstrated good discrimination in both male ($c = 0.83$) and female ($c = 0.85$) patient models. The empirical validity of the ORT was also demonstrated, as 94.4% of individuals rated as "low risk" on the ORT did not display any aberrant drug behaviors, whereas

90.9% of "high risk" individuals had at least one aberrant drug-related behavior (Webster & Webster, 2005).

The Diagnosis, Intractability, Risk, Efficacy (D.I.R.E.) tool was designed as a measure to predict medication compliance and treatment efficacy for chronic non-cancer pain patients already receiving long-term opioid therapy, or who are being considered for such treatment (Belgrade, Schamber, & Lindgren, 2006). D.I.R.E. is a 4-factor, 7-item scale, with each item scored from 1 to 3 and higher scores indicating better treatment prognosis. The total score provides a dichotomous indicator of patients who are not good candidates for long-term opioid therapy (total score from 7 to 13) and those patients who are good candidates for long-term opioid treatment (total item score from 14 to 21). The D.I.R.E. scale demonstrated good internal consistency ($\alpha = 0.80$) and reliability (ICC = 0.90, interrater) (ICC = 0.95, intrarater). The sensitivity and specificity of the D.I.R.E. score for predicting treatment compliance (94%/87%), medication efficacy (81%/76%), and final disposition (continue or stop opioids at last clinical visit) (86%/73%) were all high (Belgrade et al., 2006).

The Pain Assessment and Documentation Tool was intended to provide a consistent tool for measuring progress in pain management treatment over time. Items that measure four domains (pain relief, patient functioning, adverse events, and drug-related behaviors) generated from addiction literature and expert consensus were field tested by 27 clinicians in a sample ($n = 388$) of chronic noncancer pain patients (Passik et al., 2004). The resulting 41-item tool was formatted for utilization as a chart note for assessment and documentation within the clinical setting of pain management.

The Addiction Behaviors Checklist (ABC) is a 20-item scale that tracks observable behaviors characteristic of addiction to prescription opioid medications within the chronic pain patient population. The screen assays for behaviors that occur both during and between clinic visits and is intended to measure changes in behaviors over time (Wu et al., 2006). The measure was validated in a sample ($n = 136$) of patients on long-term opioid treatment. The measure demonstrated good interrater reliability (0.94, $P < 0.01$) and content validity; mean ABC total scores were significantly higher for inappropriate medication users, $M = 5.31$ (SD = 2.96), compared to appropriate medication users mean scores, $M = 1$ (SD = 1.27), $t (16) = 5.75$, $P < 0.01$. A cutoff score of ≥ 3 demonstrated optimal sensitivity (87.5%) and specificity (86.14%).

> ▶ **KEY POINT**
>
> A standardized opioid risk assessment plan should be implemented and applied for every patient receiving opioid therapy.

The Screener to Predict Opiate Misuse in Chronic Pain Patients (SOAPP-R) is a revised 24-item scale that predicts aberrant medication-related behaviors among individuals with chronic pain. Each item on the scale can be answered from 0 (never) to 4 (very often) and the individual item scores are summed to produce a total scale score (Butler, Fernandez, Benoit, Budman, & Jamison, 2008). The SOAPP-R was initially validated in a sample ($n = 284$) of chronic pain patients on long-term opioid therapy. The scale demonstrated good test–retest reliability (ICC = 0.92) and internal consistency ($\alpha = 0.88$). The sensitivity (81%) and specificity (68%) at a cutoff score of 18 were good (AUC = 0.81; 95% CI: 0.75-0.89, $P < 0.001$). The SOAPP-R was cross-validated in a sample ($n = 302$) of chronic noncancer pain patients followed up for 5 months (Butler, Budman, Fernandez, Fanciullo, & Jamison, 2009). The reliability and predictive validity of the scale, measured by the area under the curve (AUC) were highly significant (ICC = 0.91; 95% CI: 0.86-0.94) (α = 0.86) (AUC = 0.74; 95% CI: 0.67-0.81, P < 0001). The sensitivity (80%) and specificity (0.52) of the scale with a cutoff score of 18 were similar to the original sample.

Pain Management in all Patients with Chronic Pain Syndromes

The screening tools discussed in the preceding section are not intended to independently diagnose the presence or absence of an SUD in a specific patient under evaluation for pain management. Rather, these measures are intended to serve as one component of a comprehensive strategy for the assessment, documentation, and treatment of comorbid SUDs in the general pain population. These practice guidelines are the result of a body of addiction and pain research that is continually evolving in response to major clinical and public health phenomena, particularly the opioid epidemic of the past two decades.

New research studies were undertaken to attempt to quantify the rates of opioid use disorders in chronic pain patients. Aggregate findings of these investigations, in the form of systematic reviews and meta-analyses, produced widely variable estimates of the prevalence of opioid use disorders in chronic pain patients on long-term opioid therapy (LOT); from 3.27% (Fishbain, Cole, Lewis, Rosomoff, & Rosomoff, 2008), between 3% and 48% (Morasco et al., 2011), to estimates of lifetime prevalence of 36% to 56% (Martell et al., 2007). These contradictory findings were the result of several methodologic factors that limited the quality of evidence in addiction and pain research. The lack of clear and unambiguous definition of terms such as "addiction," "substance abuse," and "substance dependence" meant that different studies were utilizing different criteria to determine which patients were experiencing addiction disease. Furthermore, these studies were almost universally retrospective rather than prospective in design and were thereby unable to show the longitudinal relationship between opioid use and addiction over time. A more recent analysis quantified the rate of opioid addiction using stringent criterion (*DSM IV* or *ICD-9* diagnostic criteria) and detected the frequency of iatrogenic opioid dependence or abuse at 4.7% (95% CI: 2.1%-10.4%) (Higgins, Smith, & Matthews, 2018). Even within this study, addiction rates were significantly different depending on the diagnostic criteria (*DSM IV* vs. *ICD-9*) used, and only 5 of the 12 studies included within the meta-analysis used longitudinal designs, severely limiting the ability to infer whether prescription opioid use preceded or was preceded by addiction in this patient population. Other research showed that opioids did not have significant safety and efficacy in treating pain lasting longer than 3 months and demonstrated that high attrition rates confounded the ability to draw positive conclusions about the efficacy and safety of opioids in the treatment of chronic pain (Furlan, Sandoval, Mailis-Gagnon, & Tunks, 2006; Noble, Tregear, Treadwell, & Schoelles, 2008). The aggregate results of the newer research on LOT for chronic noncancer pain led to an increasing awareness of the increased risks of addiction with chronic opioid administration, with an attendant shift in practice guidelines that no longer advocated for opioids as first-line treatment for chronic pain syndromes.

The past decade has seen the creation of numerous evidence-based practice guidelines for the management of chronic pain that have deemphasized the role of opioid monotherapy in favor of multimodal treatment approaches incorporating pharmacologic and nonpharmacologic treatments. The CDC disseminated a set of evidence-based practice guidelines for prescribing opioids for chronic pain. The guidelines provide 12 recommendations to guide the use of opioids in clinical practice. The guidelines specifically assert that nonopioid therapy is the preferred treatment for chronic pain (CDC, 2016). Specific recommendations include:

> opioids should only be used when benefits for pain and function are expected to outweigh risks, Prior to initiating opioid therapy clinicians and patients should establish treatment goals and circumstances where opioids would be discontinued, prescribe the lowest effect dosage of opioids, carefully assess risks and benefits when considering increasing dosage to 50 morphine milligram equivalents (MME) or more per day, avoid concurrent opioid and benzodiazepine treatment whenever possible, Evaluate benefits and harms of continuing opioid therapy at least every 3 months and review prescription drug monitoring program data, clinicians should offer or refer evidence based treatment, such as medically assisted treatment with buprenorphine or methadone to patients with opioid use disorders. (CDC, 2016)

The CDC guidelines provide detailed instructions for ensuring safety and efficacy when treating chronic pain with or without opioids and are a valuable resource for practitioners working with pain patients or SUDs. The CDC guidelines are in agreement with a treatment paradigm for chronic pain that has come to be known as "universal precautions." In the same way that patient safety and infection control is ensured by treating all body fluids as potentially infectious, universal precautions in chronic pain treatment ensure patient safety by providing a common set of assessment and diagnostic tools that address addiction risk in any patient being considered for long-term opioid treatment (Webster & Fine, 2010), Some of the components of the recommended universal precautions include: use of instruments that assess risk of addiction (discussed previously), use of treatment contracts in opioid prescribing, implementation of urinalysis testing for drug metabolites, consultation of a statewide prescription drug monitoring program, the utilization of a multimodal treatment approach to chronic pain that relies upon adjunctive (nonopioid) analgesics and nonpharmacologic treatment interventions and is "opioid sparing," and collaboration with addiction treatment providers in providing coordinated services to individuals with comorbid SUDs and pain. A treatment contract is a written document that specifies the conditions of treatment and provides remedies for any potential eventualities (such as treatment failure or illicit drug use) that the practitioner and patient agree upon at the beginning of the treatment period. Because self-report assessment measures and treatment contracts are reliant on subjective measures of patient self-report and clinician judgment, and patients may be motivated to conceal substance use information they feel could endanger the treatment relationship, a formal procedure for urinalysis of drug metabolites is highly recommended when patients are prescribed opioids for chronic pain. Best practices for urinalysis testing have been created, and these provide guidelines for practitioners (selection of drugs to screen for the potential for false positives and false negatives with immunoassays, and the importance of discussing positive findings for illicit drugs with patients and using confirmatory testing with a gas chromatograph/liquid spectrometry assay) (Argoff et al., 2018). Prescription drug monitoring programs are statewide databases of opioid prescriptions that allow a practitioner to see if a patient is retrieving opioid prescriptions from multiple providers, a behavior that is possibly suggestive of addiction or drug diversion that requires further investigation. An important aspect of this treatment approach is that results that are suggestive of the potential presence of an opioid use disorder (such as positive illicit drugs on urine screening or multiple opioid prescriptions from multiple providers in the prescription monitoring program (PMP) database) should not be used as grounds for dismissing a patient from treatment, but must be used as an opportunity for coordinated care involving referral and collaboration with addiction treatment providers. The research evidence indicates that effective management of comorbid pain and addiction disease requires simultaneous treatment of both the patient's pain and addiction pathology (Compton, 2011; Oliver et al., 2012). The practice guidelines provide a framework for ensuring the optimal level of safety and efficacy in chronic pain management. When a patient is identified with current or a history of SUDs, there are specific guidelines that apply safe and effective care provision.

Pain Management in Patients with Comorbid SUDs

When treating a patient who has comorbid pain and SUDs, the use of broader guidelines from the chronic pain domain (such as the CDC guidelines and the universal precautions) provides a good foundation to which a greater level of vigilance and caregiver coordination is added. It is important that nurse practitioners working in the pain management field understand the pharmacologic and non-pharmacologic treatment interventions that are used in addiction medicine. The primary pharmacologic intervention for opioid use disorders with a strong evidence base is medication-assisted treatment (MAT) with either opioid agonist or opioid antagonist medications. Methadone is a full agonist of the Mu Opioid Receptor (MOR) that is given as a daily maintenance medication for opioid addiction. The long half-life of methadone provides a steady serum level that prevents withdrawal symptoms without producing the euphoria of a strong MOR agonist (such as morphine or heroin). Buprenorphine is a partial MOR agonist and an antagonist at the Kappa Opioid Receptor (KOR). It is typically given as a daily sublingual dosage and has less potent psychological effects than methadone because of its partial agonist properties, while some evidence that antagonism of the KOR receptor is also involved in decreasing opioid-induced hyperalgesia contributes to its therapeutic effect. Buprenorphine that is used for MAT therapy is in a mixed formulation with the MOR antagonist naloxone (Suboxone), which deters misuse of the drug for euphoric effects. The primary difference in the treatment infrastructure for methadone and Suboxone (buprenorphine: naloxone) is that methadone can only be dispensed from federally licensed specialty clinics, whereas Suboxone can

> ▶ **KEY POINT**
>
> Medication-assisted treatment is used to treat the underlying neurobiologic disease of addiction and is not dosed to treat pain.

be prescribed by a physician in primary practice who obtains a certification. The decision to use methadone or Suboxone is largely determined by availability and patient preference. Although there is mixed evidence related to efficacy, methadone seems to produce better treatment retention rates (Eder et al., 1998; Fischer et al., 1999; Hser et al., 2016; Kosten, Schottenfeld, Ziedonis, & Falcioni, 1993; Pinto et al., 2010), whereas Suboxone patients who remain in treatment have been shown to have a lower frequency of illicit drug use in some studies (Curcio, Franco, Topa, Baldassarre, & Gruppo Responsabili UO Sert T, 2011; Fischer et al., 1999; Pinto et al., 2010). The other medication used in MAT therapy is naltrexone, which is a longer acting formulation of the MOR antagonist naloxone (Narcan). Naltrexone can be taken orally, but has very low success rates. An injectable long-lasting depot formulation of naltrexone (Vivitrol), given on a monthly basis, has been developed more recently, and has been shown to have comparable efficacy to methadone and Suboxone. Understanding the pharmacology of the different MAT therapies is important because they have important effects on pain in patients taking MAT therapy.

The provision of pain management in patients with comorbid SUDs necessarily involves the coordinated implementation of treatment for both the patient's pain as well as the patient's addiction pathology. To a large extent, the shape this treatment will take depends on both the severity of the patient's pain and their location on the spectrum from active addiction to recovery (either through abstinence or with MAT therapy). The CDC guidelines discourage the use of opioids in chronic pain patients and this would seem to be wise when dealing with patients with opioid or other SUDs, owing to the inherent risk of relapse, overdose, and death that can result from exposure to opioids. Determining the best course of action, whether the decision to use opioids is made or not, should always involve consultation with the patient and with their addiction treatment providers. An important consideration when working with patients potentially at risk of opioid overdose, such as individuals with a history of substance use or individuals on high-dose opiate analgesia, is the possibility of providing these at-risk patients with the opiate overdose reversal drug naloxone (Narcan). Narcan is a powerful antagonist of the Mu opiate receptor that can be safely used to reverse an opiate/opioid overdose. Narcan is available to the public without a prescription in most states and covered by many insurance plans (some public health assistance programs also provide Narcan at reduced cost, National Institute on Drug Abuse, National Institutes of Health, & U.S. Department of Health and Human Services, 2017). Narcan training involves teaching individuals to recognize the signs of an overdose, notify 911, and administer Narcan while performing rescue breathing. It is important to note that individuals cannot administer Narcan to themselves to reverse an overdose, and follow-up medical care is essential, as the effect of Narcan can wear off before opioids clear the system, putting people back into an overdose. Also, multiple doses of Narcan may be necessary if a patient has ingested powerful MOR agonists (such as fentanyl). Narcan is a safe and effective harm-reduction strategy and it should be offered to individuals at high overdose risk or their family members and friends. The following section summarizes treatment guidelines for acute and chronic pain in patients with SUDs.

Acute Pain

When a patient is receiving MAT therapy, this will affect their opioid tolerance and consultation with the addiction provider to determine appropriate medication changes is needed. Methadone patients have both a high opioid tolerance (which decreases the effect of opioid analgesia) and an increased risk of overdose (because of the long half-life of methadone). Buprenorphine has less of an overdose risk, but the high affinity of the drug for the MOR receptor as well as its limited activation of the receptor could potentially interfere with opioid analgesia in situations where significant pain is expected (CDC, 2016). Some research has recommended temporary discontinuation of buprenorphine MAT during an acute pain episode (such as a surgery or delivery), although other research suggests that patient outcomes are better if MAT treatment is continued during these acute pain conditions (Höflich et al., 2011; Jones et al., 2009). Individuals on naltrexone are of particular concern in an acute pain situation, as the strong antagonism of the MOR by the drug can completely block the analgesic effects of opioid painkillers (Vickers & Jolly, 2006). An alternative strategy in all of these situations involves the use of multimodal pharmacology (nonsteroidal anti-inflammatory drugs [NSAIDs], local anesthetics, clonidine, ketamine), which act on multiple pain pathways and limit or remove the need for opioid treatment during acute pain (surgery or childbirth) (Loftus et al., 2010). Regardless of the choice, close consultation with the patient, the addiction treatment provider, and the pain management team is critically important. A patient in recovery may choose to forego opioid treatment or may elect to receive opioids and increase the level of addiction treatment (MAT therapy, psychosocial/counseling, AA/NA fellowship) to decrease their risk of relapse.

> ▶ **KEY POINT**
>
> When treating pain in patients on medication-assisted treatment, the use of multimodal therapies can help to relieve pain, improve function, and prevent relapse.

Chronic Pain

Given the significant risks associated with long-term opioid use and the lack of evidence for safety and efficacy of opioids in chronic pain, the CDC does not recommend them as a primary treatment for chronic pain. As stated previously, the practice recommendations for a person in addiction or recovery would focus on multimodal pain management. This treatment involves the use of multiple non-opioid medications that target multiple pain pathways (NSAIDs, acetaminophen, gabapentin/pregabalin, alpha blockers [clonidine], anticonvulsants, local anesthetics, tricyclic antidepressants) that have demonstrated efficacy in managing chronic pain. Multimodal treatment would likely also involve evidence-based nonpharmacologic interventions that have demonstrated efficacy in treating both pain and addiction. Validated treatments include cognitive behavioral therapy (mindfulness and Acceptance and Commitment Therapy) (Garland et al., 2014; Khusid & Vythilingam, 2016; Smallwood, Potter, & Robin, 2016), acupuncture, massage, biofeedback, physical therapy, and chiropractic treatment (Tick et al., 2018). Should opioid medications be necessary, they should be given according to the CDC guidelines, with increased monitoring for adverse outcomes and coordination with addiction treatment and recovery resources. Benzodiazepine treatment should be avoided because of the significant risk of overdose and respiratory depression (Reisfield & Webster, 2013).

REFERENCES

Argoff, C. E., Alford, D. P., Fudin, J., Adler, J. A., Bair, M. J., Dart, R. C., . . . Webster, L. R. (2018). Rational urine drug monitoring in patients receiving opioids for chronic pain: Consensus recommendations. *Pain Medicine, 19*(1), 97–117. Retrieved from http://ezproxy.lib.uconn.edu/login?url=https://search.ebscohost.com/login.aspx?direct=true&db=sph&AN=127505006&site=ehost-live

Belgrade, M. J., Schamber, C. D., & Lindgren, B. R. (2006). The DIRE score: Predicting outcomes of opioid prescribing for chronic pain. *The Journal of Pain, 7*(9), 671–681. doi:10.1016/j.jpain.2006.03.001

Butler, S. F., Budman, S. H., Fanciullo, G. J., & Jamison, R. N. (2010). Cross validation of the current opioid misuse measure to monitor chronic pain patients on opioid therapy. *The Clinical Journal of Pain, 26*(9), 770–776. doi:10.1097/AJP.0b013e3181f195ba

Butler, S. F., Budman, S. H., Fernandez, K. C., Fanciullo, G. J., & Jamison, R. N. (2009). Cross-validation of a screener to predict opioid misuse in chronic pain patients (SOAPP-R). *Journal of Addiction Medicine, 3*(2), 66–73. doi:10.1097/ADM.0b013e31818e41da

Butler, S. F., Budman, S. H., Fernandez, K. C., Houle, B., Benoit, C., Katz, N., & Jamison, R. N. (2007). Development and validation of the current opioid misuse measure. *Pain, 130*(1), 144–156. doi:10.1016/j.pain.2007.01.014

Butler, S. F., Fernadzez, K., Benoit, C., Budman, S. H. & Jamison, R. N. (2008). Validation of the revised Screener and Opioid Assessment for Patients with Pain (SOAPP-R). *Journal of Pain, 9*(4), 360–372. doi:10.1016/j.jpain.2007.11.014

Centers for Disease Control and Prevention. (2011). Vital signs: Overdoses of prescription opioid pain relievers—United States, 1999–2008. *Morbidity and Mortality Weekly Report, 60*(43), 1487–1492.

Centers for Disease Control and Prevention. (2016). CDC guideline for prescribing opioids for chronic pain—United States, 2016. *MMWR Recommendations and Reports, 65*(No. RR-1), 1–49. doi:10.15585/mmwr.rr6501e1

Compton, P. (2011). Treating chronic pain with prescription opioids in the substance abuser: Relapse prevention and management. *Journal of Addictions Nursing, 22*(1), 39–45. doi:10.3109/10884602.2010.545092

Curcio, F., Franco, T., Topa, M., Baldassarre, C., & Gruppo Responsabili UO Sert T. (2011). Buprenorphine/naloxone versus methadone in opioid dependence: A longitudinal survey. *European Review for Medical and Pharmacological Sciences, 15*(8), 871–874.

Eder, H., Fischer, G., Gombas, W., Jagsch, R., Stuhlinger, G., & Kasper, S. (1998). Comparison of buprenorphine and methadone maintenance in opiate addicts. *European Addiction Research, 4*(Suppl. 1), 3–7. doi:10.1159/000052034

Fischer, G., Gombas, W., Eder, H., Jagsch, R., Peternell, A., Stuhlinger, G., . . . Kasper, S. (1999). Buprenorphine versus methadone maintenance for the treatment of opioid dependence. *Addiction, 94*(9), 1337–1347.

Fishbain, D. A., Cole, B., Lewis, J., Rosomoff, H. L., & Rosomoff, R. S. (2008). What percentage of chronic nonmalignant pain patients exposed to chronic opioid analgesic therapy develop abuse/addiction and/or aberrant drug-related behaviors? A structured evidence-based review. *Pain Medicine, 9*(4), 444–459. doi:10.1111/j.1526-4637.2007.00370.x

Furlan, A. D., Sandoval, J. A., Mailis-Gagnon, A., & Tunks, E. (2006). Opioids for chronic noncancer pain: A meta-analysis of effectiveness and side effects. *CMAJ: Canadian Medical Association Journal, 174*(11), 1589–1594. Retrieved from http://ezproxy.lib.uconn.edu/login?url=https://search.ebscohost.com/login.aspx?direct=true&db=cmedm&AN=16717269&site=ehost-live

Garland, E. L., Froeliger, B., Williams, J. M., Manusov, E. G., Kelly, A., & Howard, M. O. (2014). Mindfulness-oriented recovery enhancement for chronic pain and prescription opioid misuse: Results from an early-stage randomized controlled trial. *Journal of Consulting & Clinical Psychology, 82*(3), 448–459. doi:10.1037/a0035798

Higgins, C., Smith, B. H., & Matthews, K. (2018). Incidence of iatrogenic opioid dependence or abuse in patients with pain who were exposed to opioid analgesic therapy: A systematic review and meta-analysis. *British Journal of Anaesthesia, 120*(6), 1335-1344.

Höflich, A. S., Langer, M., Jagsch, R., Bäwert, A., Winklbaur, B., Fischer, G., . . . Unger, A. (2012). Peripartum pain management in opioid dependent women. *European Journal of Pain, 16*(4), 574–584. doi:10.1016/j.ejpain.2011.08.008

Holmes, C. P., Gatchel, R. J., Adams, L. L., Stowell, A. W., Hatten, A., Noe, C., & Lou, L. (2006). An opioid screening instrument: Long-term evaluation of the utility of the pain medication questionnaire. *Pain Practice, 6*(2), 74–88. doi:10.1111/j.1533-2500.2006.00067.x

Hser, Y. I., Evans, E., Huang, D., Weiss, R., Saxon, A., Carroll, K. M., . . . Ling, W. (2016). Long-term outcomes after randomization to buprenorphine/naloxone versus methadone in a multi-site trial. *Addiction, 111*(4), 695–705. doi:10.1111/add.13238

Jones, H. E., O'Grady, K., Dahne, J., Johnson, R., Lemoine, L., Milio, L., . . . Selby, P. (2009). Management of acute postpartum pain in patients maintained on methadone or buprenorphine during pregnancy. *American Journal of Drug & Alcohol Abuse, 35*(3), 151–156. doi:10.1080/00952990902825413

Khusid, M. A., & Vythilingam, M. (2016). The emerging role of mindfulness meditation as effective self-management strategy, part 2: Clinical implications for chronic pain, substance misuse, and insomnia. *Military Medicine, 181*(9), 969–975. doi:10.7205/MILMED-D-14-00678

Kosten, T. R., Schottenfeld, R., Ziedonis, D., & Falcioni, J. (1993). Buprenorphine versus methadone maintenance for opioid dependence. *Journal of Nervous and Mental Disease, 181*(6), 358–364.

Loftus, R. W., Yeager, M. P., Clark, J. A., Brown, J. R., Abdu, W. A., Sengupta, D. K., & Beach, M. L. (2010). Intraoperative ketamine reduces perioperative opiate consumption in opiate-dependent patients with chronic back pain undergoing back surgery. *Anesthesiology, 113*(3), 639–646. doi:10.1097/ALN.0b013e3181e90914

Martell, B. A., O'Connor, P. G., Kerns, R. D., Becker, W., Morales, K. H., Kosten, T. R., & Fiellin, D. A. (2007). Systematic review: Opioid treatment for chronic back pain: Prevalence, efficacy, and association with addiction. *Annals of Internal Medicine, 146*, 116–127.

Morasco, B. J., Gritzner, S., Lewis, L., Oldham, R., Turk, D. C., & Dobscha, S. K. (2011). Systematic review of prevalence, correlates, and treatment outcomes for chronic non-cancer pain in patients with comorbid substance use disorder. *Pain, 152*(3), 488–497. doi:10.1016/j.pain.2010.10.009

National Center for Health Statistics. (2018). *Overdose death rates 1999–2017.* Retrieved from https://www.drugabuse.gov/related-topics/trends-statistics/overdose-death-rates

National Institute on Drug Abuse, National Institutes of Health, & U.S. Department of Health and Human Services. (2017). *Naloxone for opioid overdose: Life-saving science.* Retrieved from https://www.drugabuse.gov/publications/naloxone-opioid-overdose-life-saving-science/naloxone-opioid-overdose-life-saving-science

National Institute on Drug Abuse, National Institutes of Health, & U.S. Department of Health and Human Services. (2018). *DrugFacts: Heroin.* Retrieved from https://www.drugabuse.gov/publications/drugfacts/heroin#ref

Noble, M., Tregear, S. J., Treadwell, J. R., & Schoelles, K. (2008). Long-term opioid therapy for chronic noncancer pain: A systematic review and meta-analysis of efficacy and safety. *Journal of Pain and Symptom Management, 35*(2), 214–228. doi:10.1016/j.jpainsymman.2007.03.015

Oliver, J., Coggins, C., Compton, P., Hagan, S., Matteliano, D., Stanton, M., . . . Turner, H. N. (2012). American society for pain management nursing position statement: Pain management in patients with substance use disorders. *Journal of Addictions Nursing, 23*(3), 210–222. doi:10.1097/JAN.0b013e318271c123

Passik, S. D., Kirsh, K. L., Whitcomb, L., Portenoy, R. K., Katz, N. P., Kleinman, L., . . . Schein, J. R. (2004). A new tool to assess and document pain outcomes in chronic pain patients receiving opioid therapy. *Clinical Therapeutics, 26*(4), 552–561. Retrieved from http://ezproxy.lib.uconn.edu/login?url=https://search.ebscohost.com/login.aspx? direct=true&db=cmedm&AN=15189752&site=ehost-live

Pinto, H., Maskrey, V., Swift, L., Rumball, D., Wagle, A., & Holland, R. (2010). The SUMMIT trial: A field comparison of buprenorphine versus methadone maintenance treatment. *Journal of Substance Abuse Treatment, 39*(4), 340–352. doi:10.1016/j.jsat.2010.07.009

Reisfield, G. M., & Webster, L. R. (2013). Benzodiazepines in long- term opioid therapy. *Pain Medicine, 14*(10), 1441–1446. doi:10.1111/pme.12236

Smallwood, R. F., Potter, J. S., & Robin, D. A. (2016). Neurophysiological mechanisms in acceptance and commitment therapy in opioid-addicted patients with chronic pain. *Psychiatry Research: Neuroimaging Section, 250*, 12–14. doi:10.1016/j.pscychresns.2016.03.001

Tick, H., Nielsen, A., Pelletier, K. R., Bonakdar, R., Simmons, S., Glick, R., . . . Zador, V. (2018). Evidence-based nonpharmacologic strategies for comprehensive pain care: The consortium pain task force white paper. *Explore: The Journal of Science & Healing, 14*(2), 177–211. doi:10.1016/j.explore.2018.02.001

Vickers, A. P., & Jolly, A. (2006). Naltrexone and problems in pain management: How to manage acute pain in people taking an opioid antagonist. *BMJ: British Medical Journal (International Edition), 332*(7534), 132–133. Retrieved from http://ezproxy.lib.uconn.edu/login?url=https://search.ebscohost.com/login .aspx?direct=true&db=rzh&AN=106324019&site=ehost-live

Volkow, N., Benveniste, H., & McLellan, A. T. (2018). Use and misuse of opioids in chronic pain. *Annual Review of Medicine, 69*(1), 451. doi:10.1146/annurev-med-011817-044739

Webster, L. R., & Fine, P. G. (2010). Approaches to improve pain relief while minimizing opioid abuse liability. *Journal of Pain, 11*(7), 602–611. doi:10.1016/j.jpain.2010.02.008

Webster, L. R., & Webster, R. M. (2005). Predicting aberrant behaviors in opioid-treated patients: Preliminary validation of the opioid risk tool. *Pain Medicine, 6*(6), 432–442. Retrieved from http://ezproxy.lib.uconn.edu/login?url=https://search.ebscohost.com/login .aspx?direct=true&db=sph&AN=18986090&site=ehost-live

Wu, S. M., Compton, P., Bolus, R., Schieffer, B., Pham, Q., Baria, A., . . . Naliboff, B. D. (2006). The addiction behaviors checklist: Validation of a new clinician-based measure of inappropriate opioid use in chronic pain. *Journal of Pain & Symptom Management, 32*(4), 342–351. doi:10.1016/j.jpainsymman.2006.05.010

Zedler, B., Xie, L., Wang, L., Joyce, A., Vick, C., Brigham, J., . . . Murrelle, L. (2015). Development of a risk index for serious prescription opioid-induced respiratory depression or overdose in veterans' health administration patients. *Pain Medicine (Malden, Mass.), 16*(8), 1566–1579. doi:10.1111/pme.12777

CHAPTER 12

SYSTEM LEVEL PAIN MANAGEMENT

Jonathan Sylvain and Seth Hagymasi

Introduction

Patient safety, improvement in quality, and standardization of care have become the major focus within healthcare systems. Currently, there is wide variability of how healthcare systems work and how they incorporate system level change. Globally, billions of dollars are spent each year in the public and private sectors on biomedical, clinical, and health research, healthcare professional training and continuing education, quality improvement, and patient safety. Despite this, healthcare systems have failed to provide cost-effective programs and services to those in the community (Grimshaw, Eccles, Lavis, Hill, & Squires, 2012).

Specifically, healthcare systems have done poorly with implementing programs to effectively treat patients who are experiencing pain. Research has demonstrated that only a third of patients on sick leave for musculoskeletal symptoms and 48% of patients presenting with low back pain (LBP) are receiving evidence-based interventions (Nilsing, Söderberg, & Öberg, 2012; Wåhlin, Ekberg, Persson, Bernfort, & Öberg, 2012). Furthermore, clinicians continue to utilize interventions that they consider to be relevant despite the lack of evidence about the effects (Bernhardsson, Öberg, Johansson, Nilsen, & Larsson, 2015).

As discussed earlier in this text, pain is one of the most common reasons for seeking medical care across all age groups (National Institutes of Health, 2016). The burden of pain on the individual, family, community, and society is often underestimated. It is estimated that 23.4 million American adults, 10.3%, experience a significant amount of pain and an estimated 126 million adults, 55.7%, have reported some type of pain in the past 3 months (Nahin, 2015).

Undertreatment of pain resulting in physiologic, psychosocial, and economic consequences continues despite targeted improvement approaches (Freburger et al., 2009; Pransky, Borkan, Young, & Cherkin, 2011).

> ▶ **KEY POINT**
>
> Pain treatment requires a multidisciplinary approach that needs to be guided by evidence supporting its use and by consideration of its cost-effectiveness and feasibility in relation to other interventions. These treatments should be multimodal in nature and most often combine pharmacologic and nonpharmacologic interventions.

Within this chapter, we will discuss: (1) the concept of system level change within the healthcare environment; (2) what system level change entails; (3) considerations when planning and implementing a system level program; (4) pros/facilitators of system level change; (5) cons/barriers of system level change; (6) a specific example of system level change within a healthcare system; and (7) physical therapy–based treatment for acute spine pain within a healthcare system.

System Level Change

Understanding of the complexity of healthcare systems has grown over the past years (Braithwaite, Clay-Williams, Nugus, & Plumb, 2013; Clay-Williams, 2012), and from an evaluation of the various systems, an emphasis on system level changes is the emerging trend (Braithwaite, Westbrook, & Travaglia, 2008). To date, the focus on system level change has been on local change, quality improvement, and patient safety initiatives, which have shown limited benefits to patients (Schouten, Hulscher, Everdingen, Huijsman, & Grol, 2008) with effect sizes of 10% to 20% at best (Grimshaw et al., 2012).

The Centers for Disease Control and Prevention defines health systems change as "a change in organizational or legislative policies or in environmental supports that encourages and channels improvement(s) in systems, community, and individual-level health outcomes" (Minta, Todd, & Jernigan, n.d.). A recent example of system level change in the healthcare setting familiar to both clinicians and patients would be the implementation of electronic medical records. Several goals of the implementation of electronic medical records were to standardize the electronic capture of patient demographics, clinical orders, and results and improving quality of care through the ease of access to patient information.

A consistent finding in clinical and health services research is the failure to translate research into practice and policy (Grol, 2001; McGlynn et al., 2003). This failure results in evidence-based practice gaps and variability in the quality of care provided within the same system and contending systems. This results in patients failing to benefit from the advances in healthcare resulting in a decreased quality of life and loss of productivity at both personal and societal levels. Furthermore, evidence demonstrates that patients routinely receive care that is not needed or that could potentially be harmful (Almeida et al., 2013; Kale, Bishop, Federman, & Keyhani, 2013; Levine, Linder, & Landon, 2016; Schuster, McGlynn, & Brook, 1998). The apparent lack of guideline adherent and evidence-informed care serves to further underscore the importance of coordination of care across disciplines within healthcare systems, which may be accomplished through system level program development.

Considerations When Planning and Implementing a System Level Program

When developing a program for patients in pain, utilizing a biopsychosocial model is of vital importance. As discussed in Chapter 1, this model provides a framework for understanding the interactions between the biologic, psychological, and sociocultural factors that impact pain. Typically, healthcare systems take on a predominantly biomedical approach in the management of patients presenting with pain (Wade & Halligan, 2004). During the developmental stages of a system level program, it will be important to keep in mind that psychological and social factors will have an impact on each individual's pain experience. It has been shown that low educational status, worry, anxiety, depression, high psychological stress, poor self-rated health, frequent use of health or social services, and concurrent pain in other areas are factors that can affect outcomes in changing each individual's pain experience (Carragee, Alamin, Miller, & Carragee, 2005; Docking et al., 2011; Hoy, Brooks, Blyth, & Buchbinder, 2010; Jarvik et al., 2005; Power, Frank, Hertzman, Schierhout, & Li, 2001).

System level changes will have a higher chance of success if a wide range of staff are involved in the design, implementation, and monitoring. From an employee perspective, work factors such as job dissatisfaction, low levels of social support in the workplace, and lack of control over job tasks also need to be taken into consideration (Bigos et al., 1991) as they may reduce employee buy-in to the program, potentially leading to its failure or ineffectiveness.

During the developmental and planning stages of programs aimed at system level changes, those involved should be aware of the complexity associated with successful design, implementation, and maintenance of such a program. Following validated guidelines during the developmental stages may enhance success. Essential areas of importance during the process are building partnerships, establishing goals, developing a plan or process, and implementing, monitoring, and evaluating the plan. Figure 12-1 highlights important aspects that should be taken into consideration during healthcare program development, implementation, and evaluation.

▍Facilitators of, and Barriers to, System Level Change

The complexity associated with successful implementation of system level change has been demonstrated within the literature and current research demonstrates that there is variability in the uptake of system-wide healthcare interventions (Braithwaite et al., 2010; Hillman et al., 2005; Landrigan et al., 2010). When developing and implementing a system level program, it is vital to have an understanding of the possible barriers to, and facilitators of, the success or failure of the program (Slade et al., 2016). Table 12-1 lists possible barriers and facilitators.

▍Implementation of System Level Change—Acute Lumbar Spine Pain

There is currently an abundance of literature supporting early access to conservative interventions such as physical therapy for those with musculoskeletal injuries, with much of this literature focusing on acute onset of LBP (Childs et al., 2015; Fritz, Childs, Wainner, & Flynn, 2012; Fritz, Magel, et al., 2015; Fritz, Kim, & Dorius, 2016). Among the benefits suggested with early access to the appropriate care are: decrease

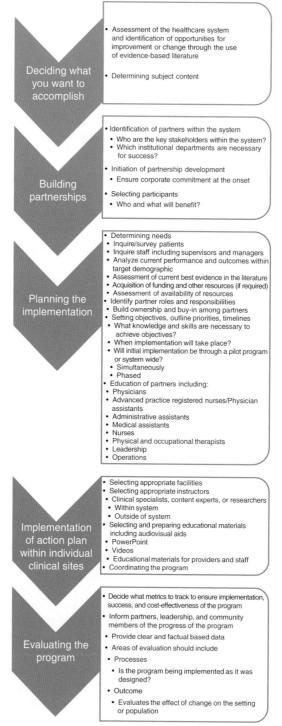

Figure 12-1. Acute lumbar spine pain program algorithm. Created by Jonathan Sylvain and Seth Hagymasi, courtesy of the University of Connecticut Musculoskeletal Institute Comprehensive Spine Center—Low Back Now Program.

Table 12–1. Facilitators and Barriers to System Level Change

Facilitators	Barriers
Included learning about the guideline through group interaction	Negative staff attitudes and beliefs
Positive staff attitudes and beliefs	Lack of or poor leadership support
Leadership support	Limited integration of guideline recommendations into organizational structures and processes
Clinical supporters of the implementation	Time and resource constraints
Teamwork and collaboration	Organizational and system level change resistance from staff
Professional association support	Referring patients who are not appropriate
Inter- and intraorganizational collaboration	Practitioners who did not believe in current best evidence despite data
Inter- and intradepartmental collaboration	Multiple clinic locations involved
	Large medical system

in healthcare costs per episode, improved recovery time, decrease in unnecessary diagnostic imaging usage, surgery, and injections (Fritz, Brennan, et al., 2015; Liu et al., 2018). Conversely, early provision of imaging modalities or opioid medication has been associated with higher LBP-related healthcare costs as well as increased risk of prolonged LBP-related disability (Webster, Bauer, Choi, Cifuentes, & Pransky, 2013). Given this information, a number of institutions have begun to enact system-wide change in the management of individuals with acute lumbar spine pain to streamline access to early and appropriate level care, reduce system-wide costs, readmissions, improve disability-related outcomes, and provide treatment supported by current literature. Figure 12-2 is an example of one such program as well as the steps taken to implement the program.

The goals of such a program can be defined in terms of both system level as well as patient centered. Examples of system level goals include: reducing emergency department readmissions for LBP, increasing access for acute back pain patients, ensuring a smooth and evidence-based escalation from conservative care (physical therapy) to specialist consultation (if necessary), and improving overall outcomes in individuals with acute LBP. Examples of patient level goals include: improvement in pain and lumbar spine active range of motion, improvement in tolerance for activities of daily living and functional activities, ability to return to work, improvement in patient reported outcome measures such as the Oswestry Disability Index and developing independence with a home exercise program for continued and future management of lumbar symptoms, as well as prevention of a reoccurrence.

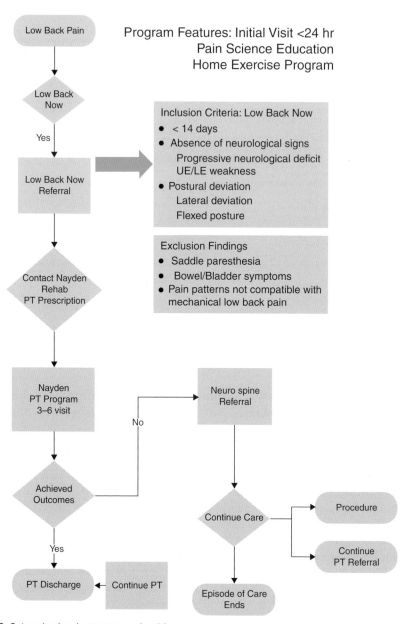

Figure 12–2. Low back pain treatment algorithm

Physical Therapy for the Treatment of Pain

Use of physical therapy as conservative management for patients with pain may include a variety of effective interventions. Traditionally, these interventions have included therapeutic and functional exercise, manual therapy, physical modalities (electrical stimulation, ultrasound, traction, application of thermal modalities, and others), as well as education interventions which may include topics such as ergonomics, lifting mechanics, pain science education, and/or recommendations for activity modifications among others. Generally, current literature supports the use of multimodal treatments potentially including components from each of these intervention categories as the most effective for a number or musculoskeletal pathologies (Cleland et al., 2009; Cleland, Fritz, Whitman, & Heath, 2007; Walker et al., 2008). More recent literature provides significant support for the inclusion of pain science education with general information regarding pain neuroscience in the treatment of patients with pain (Louw, Zimney, Puentedura, & Diener, 2016; Moseley, Nicholas, & Hodges, 2004; Nijs et al., 2017). This education provides patients with foundational information regarding the biologic function and source of pain generation, with the goal of diminishing kinesiophobia, reducing nervous system sensitivity, resulting in an increase in the willingness of the patient to participate in graded physical activity. This graded activity in turn serves to further diminish nervous system sensitivity and potentially pain and/or improve functional status despite the presence of nonharmful pain responses (Nijs, Girbe, Lundberg, Malfliet, & Sterling, 2015).

It has been proposed that although the individual effect sizes of each of these available interventions are relatively small, the combined effect may serve to reduce pain and restore function (Hancock & Hill, 2016; Keller, Hayden, Bombardier, & van Tulder, 2007). In particular, exercise activity, manual therapy including joint mobilization or manipulation, soft tissue mobilization, and pain education are recommended as interventions useful in the modulation of pain responses in patients with both acute and chronic pain (Giles & Muller, 2003; Nijs et al., 2015; Rainville, Hartigan, Jouve, & Martinez, 2004). It is generally accepted that exercise activity, when performed in the appropriate intensity, will promote the release of endogenous opioids, potentially helping to regulate pain (Lima, Abner, & Sluka, 2017). Manual therapy mechanisms of action in modulation of pain and restoration of function are somewhat less well defined, despite extensive research in this area. Current evidence suggests manual therapy interventions modulate pain largely through nonmechanical mechanisms with their effects being neurophysiologic and at the cortical level (Bialosky et al., 2018).

In recent years, there has been an attempt in physical therapy to establish a number of diagnostic, prognostic, and interventional clinical prediction rules (CPRs) in an effort to both standardize practice patterns as well as improve patient outcomes through identification of homogenous patient subgroups. Of those derived and validated through randomized controlled studies, one relates very closely to the efforts made by a number of institutions in the efforts to implement system level changes, such as in the "Low Back Now" program described previously in this chapter. Individuals presenting with LBP of less than 16 days duration, hip internal rotation of more than 35°, Fear Avoidance Belief Questionnaire (work subscale) score of lesser than 19, no symptoms distal to the knee, and hypomobility upon segmental assessment of the lumbar spine have been exhibited in multiple studies as likely to benefit from lumbar manipulation (Childs et al., 2004; Flynn et al., 2002). More pragmatically, a simpler, two-factor guideline has been suggested as well, including only acute onset (duration <16 days) and no symptoms distal to the knee as appropriate for screening and guidance of interventions (Fritz, Childs, & Flynn, 2005). Literature such as this reinforces the benefit of early identification, referral, and access to physical therapy, requiring system-wide coordination and education across disciplines. However, additional research needs to be performed to further validate findings, as found within the aforementioned CPRs, so that they are transferable to a broad spectrum of patients. CPRs are derivation studies in the initial steps of development of clinical decision rules and require follow-up studies in diverse areas with different populations and different clinicians in order to be validated.

Conclusion

Globally, healthcare systems are under tremendous pressure with regard to efficiency, safety, and economic feasibility. Healthcare systems need to continually evaluate their organizational and environmental structures, policies, and procedures with the aim of providing appropriate, effective, and evidence-based care to the communities that they serve.

System level changes have a higher chance of improving patient outcomes if a wide range of staff are involved in the design, implementation, and monitoring of large-scale interventions. Changing the culture of a healthcare system takes time, patience, trial and error, and continual evaluation to ensure implementation, success, and cost-effectiveness of the program. During the implementation, it is important to keep in mind that clinical areas will adopt changes at varying paces and educational programs will have diverse effects on different groups and services within the system. Therefore, it is vitally important to have an in-depth understanding of the current evidence in implementing system level changes as well as have a guideline to follow (see Figure 12-1).

Conservative, noninvasive treatment approaches such as physical therapy can play a large role in the management of patients with pain complaints. The utilization of multimodal treatment approaches within physical therapy, including education, manual, and movement-based interventions as part of an interdisciplinary treatment team, is consistent with current guidelines and evidence-based treatment approaches. Although challenges continue to exist, this may be accomplished in part through programmatic changes at the system level such as the "Low Back Now" program illustrated earlier in this chapter.

REFERENCES

Almeida, C. M., Rodriguez, M. A., Skootsky, S., Pregler, J., Steers, N., & Wenger, N. S. (2013). Cervical cancer screening overuse and underuse: Patient and physician factors. *American Journal of Managed Care, 19*(6), 482–489.

Bernhardsson, S., Öberg, B., Johansson, K., Nilsen, P., & Larsson, M. E. (2015). Clinical practice in line with evidence? A survey among primary care physiotherapists in western Sweden. *Journal of Evaluation in Clinical Practice, 21*, 1169–1177.

Bialosky, J. E., Beneciuk, J. M., Bishop, M. D., Coronado, R. A., Penza, C. W., Simon, C. B., & George, S. Z. (2018). Unraveling the mechanisms of manual therapy: Modeling an approach. *Journal Orthopaedic and Sports Physical Therapy, 48*(1), 8–18.

Bigos, S. J., Battié, M. C., Spengler, D. M., Fisher, L. D., Fordyce, W. E., Hansson, T. H., . . . Wortley, M. D. (1991). A prospective study of work perceptions and psychosocial factors affecting the report of back injury. *Spine, 16*, 1–6.

Braithwaite, J., Westbrook, M., & Travaglia, J. (2008). Attitudes toward the large-scale implementation of an incident reporting system. *International Journal for Quality in Health Care, 20*, 184–191.

Braithwaite, J., Clay-Williams, R., Nugus, P., & Plumb, J. (2013). Health care as a complex adaptive system. In E. Hollnagel, J. Braithwaite, & R. Wears (Eds.), *Resilient health care* (pp. 57–73). Surrey, UK: Ashgate.

Braithwaite, J., Greenfield, D., Westbrook, J., Pawsey, M., Westbrook, M., Gibberd, R., . . . Lancaster, J. (2010). Health service accreditation as a predictor of clinical and organisational performance: A blinded, random, stratified study. *Quality and Safety in Health Care, 19*(1), 14–21.

Carragee, E. J., Alamin, T. F., Miller, J. L., & Carragee, J. M. (2005). Discographic, MRI and psychosocial determinants of low back pain disability and remission. *Spine Journal, 5*, 24–35.

Childs, J. D., Fritz, J. M., Flynn, T. W., Irrgang, J. J., Johnson, K. K., Majkowski, G. R., & Delitto, A. (2004). A clinical prediction rule to identify patients with low back pain most likely to benefit from spinal manipulation: A validation study. *Annals of Internal Medicine, 141*(12), 920–928.

Childs, J. D., Fritz, J. M., Wu, S. S., Flynn, T. W., Wainner, R. S., Robertson, E. K., . . . George, S. Z. (2015). Implications of early and guideline adherent physical therapy for low back pain on utilization and costs. *BMC Health Services Research, 15*, 150.

Clay-Williams, R. (2012). Restructuring and the resilient organisation: Implications for health care. In E. Hollnagel, J. Braithwaite, & R. Wears (Eds.), *Resilient health care* (pp. 123-133). Surrey, UK: Ashgate Publishing Limited.

Cleland, J. A., Fritz, J. M., Whitman, J. M., & Heath, R. (2007). Predictors of short-term outcome in people with a clinical diagnosis of cervical radiculopathy. *Physical Therapy, 87*(12), 1619–1632.

Cleland, J. A., Abbott, J. H., Kidd, M. O., Stockwell, S., Cheney, S., Gerrard, D. F., & Flynn, T. W. (2009). Manual physical therapy and exercise versus electrophysical agents and exercise in the management of plantar heel pain: A multicenter randomized clinical trial. *Journal Orthopaedic and Sports Physical Therapy, 39*(8), 573–585.

Docking, R. E., Fleming, J., Brayne, C., Zhao, J., Macfarlane, G. J., Jones, G. T., & Cambridge City Over-75s Cohort Study collaboration. (2011). Epidemiology of back pain in older adults: Prevalence and risk factors for back pain onset. *Rheumatology (Oxford), 50*, 1645–1653.

Flynn, T., Fritz, J., Whitman, J., Wainner, R., Magel, J., Rendeiro, D., . . . Allison, S. (2002). A clinical prediction rule for classifying patients with low back pain who demonstrate short-term improvement with spinal manipulation. *Spine, 27*(24), 2835–2843.

Freburger, J. K., Holmes, G. M., Agans, R. P., Jackman, A. M., Darter, J. D., Wallace, A. S., . . . Carey, T. S. (2009). The rising prevalence of chronic low back pain. *Archives of Internal Medicine, 169*(3), 251–258.

Fritz, J. M., Childs, J. D., & Flynn, T. W. (2005). Pragmatic application of a clinical prediction rule in primary care to identify patients with low back pain with a good prognosis following a brief spinal manipulation intervention. *BMC Family Practice, 6*(1), 29.

Fritz, J. M., Childs, J. D., Wainner, R. S., & Flynn, T. W. (2012). Primary care referral of patients with low back pain to physical therapy: Impact on future health care utilization and costs. *Spine, 37*(25), 2114–2121.

Fritz, J. M., Brennan, G. P., & Hunter, S. J. (2015). Physical therapy or advanced imaging as first management strategy following a new consultation for low back pain in primary care: Associations with future health care utilization and charges. *Health Services Research, 50*(6), 1927–1940.

Fritz, J. M., Magel, J. S., McFadden, M., Asche, C., Thackeray, A., Meier, W., & Brennan, G. (2015). Early physical therapy vs usual care in patients with recent-onset low back pain: A randomized clinical trial. *JAMA, 314*(14), 1459–1467.

Fritz, J. M., Kim, J., & Dorius, J. (2016). Importance of the type of provider seen to begin health care for a new episode low back pain: Associations with future utilizations and costs. *Journal of Evaluation in Clinical Practice, 22*(2), 247–252.

Giles, L. G. F., & Muller, R. (2003). A randomized clinical trial comparing medication, acupuncture, and spinal manipulation. *Spine, 28*(14), 1490–1503.

Grimshaw, J. M., Eccles, M. P., Lavis, J. N., Hill, S. J., & Squires, J. E. (2012). Knowledge translation of research findings. *Implementation Science, 7*, 50. doi:10.1186/1748-5908-7-50

Grol, R. (2001). Successes and failures in the implementation of evidence-based guidelines for clinical practice. *Medical Care, 39*, II46–II54.

Hancock, M. J., & Hill, J. C. (2016). Are small effects for back pain interventions really surprising? *Journal of Orthopedic & Sports Physical Therapy, 46*(5), 317–319.

Hillman, K., Chen, J., Cretikos, M., Bellomo, R., Brown, D., Doig, G., . . . Flabouris, A. (2005). Introduction of the medical emergency team (MET) system: A cluster-randomised controlled trial. *Lancet, 365*(9477), 2091–2097.

Hoy, D., Brooks, P., Blyth, F., & Buchbinder, R. (2010). The epidemiology of low back pain. *Best Practice and Research. Clinical Rheumatology, 24*, 769–781.

Jarvik, J. G., Hollingworth, W., Heagerty, P. J., Haynor, D. R., Boyko, E. J., & Deyo, R. A. (2005). Three-year incidence of low back pain in an initially asymptomatic cohort: clinical and imaging risk factors. *Spine, 30*, 1541–1548.

Kale, M. S., Bishop, T. F., Federman, A. D., & Keyhani, S. (2013). Trends in the overuse of ambulatory health care services in the United States. *JAMA Internal Medicine, 173*(2), 142–148. doi:10.1001/2013.jamainternmed.1022

Keller, A., Hayden, J., Bombardier, C., & van Tulder, M. (2007). Effect sizes of non-surgical treatments of non-specific low-back pain. *European Spine Journal, 16*(11), 1776–1788.

Landrigan, C. P., Parry, G. J., Bones, C. B., Hackbarth, A. D., Goldmann, D. A., & Sharek, P. J. (2010). Temporal trends in rates of patient harm resulting from medical care. *New England Journal of Medicine, 363*(22), 2124–2134.

Levine, D. M., Linder, J. A., & Landon, B. E. (2016). The quality of outpatient care delivered to adults in the United States, 2002 to 2013. *JAMA Internal Medicine, 176*(12), 1778–1790. doi:10.1001/jamainternmed.2016.6217

Lima, L. V., Abner, T. S. S., & Sluka, K. A. (2017). Does exercise increase or decrease pain? Central mechanisms underlying these two phenomena. *Journal of Physiology, 595*(13), 4141–4150.

Liu, X., Hanney, W. J., Masaracchio, M., Kolber, M. J., Zhao, M., Spaulding, A. C., & Gabriel, M. H. (2018). Immediate physical therapy initiation in patients with acute low back pain is associated with a reduction in downstream health care utilization and costs. *Physical Therapy, 98*(5), 336–347.

Louw, A., Zimney, K., Puentedura, E. J., & Diener, I. (2016). The efficacy of pain neuroscience education in musculoskeletal pain: A systematic review of the literature. *Physiotherapy Theory and Practice, 32*(5), 332–355.

McGlynn, E. A., Asch, S. M., Adams, J., Keesey, J., Hicks, J., DeCristofaro, A., & Kerr, E. A. (2003). The quality of health care delivered to adults in the United States. *New England Journal of Medicine, 348*, 2635–2645.

Minta, B., Todd, R., & Jernigan, J. (n.d.). *A guide to facilitating health system change.* Retrieved from https://www.cdc.gov/dhdsp/programs/spha/docs/guide_facilitating_hs_change.pdf

Moseley, G. L., Nicholas, M. K., & Hodges, P. W. (2004). A randomized controlled trial of intensive neurophysiology education in chronic low back pain. *Clinical Journal of Pain, 20*, 324–330.

Nahin, R. (2015). Estimates of pain prevalence and severity in adults: United States, 2012. *Journal of Pain, 16*(8), 769–780. doi:10.1016/j.jpain.2015.05.002

National Institutes of Health. (2016). *National pain strategy, a comprehensive population health-level strategy for pain.* Washington, DC: Department of Health and Human Services.

Nijs, J., Girbe, E. L., Lundberg, M., Malfliet, A., & Sterling, M. (2015). Exercise therapy for chronic musculoskeletal pain: Innovation by altering pain memories. *Manual Therapy, 20,* 216–220.

Nijs, J., Clark, J., Malfliet, A., Ickmans, K., Voogt, L., Don, S., . . . Dankaerts, W. (2017). In the spine or in the brain? Recent advances in pain neuroscience applied in the intervention for low back pain. *Clinical and Experimental Rheumatology, 35*(Suppl. 107), S108–S115.

Nilsing, E., Söderberg, E., & Öberg, B. (2012). Sickness certificates in Sweden: Did the new guidelines improve their quality? *BMC Public Health, 12,* 907.

Power, C., Frank, J., Hertzman, C., Schierhout, G., & Li, L. (2001). Predictors of low back pain onset in a prospective British study. *American Journal of Public Health, 91,* 1671–1678.

Pransky, G., Borkan, J. M., Young, A., & Cherkin, D. (2011). Are we making progress? *Spine, 36,* 1608–1614.

Rainville, J., Hartigan, C., Jouve, C., & Martinez, E. (2004). The influence of intense exercise-based physical therapy program on back pain anticipated before and induced by physical activities. *The Spine Journal, 4,* 176–183.

Schouten, L. M., Hulscher, M. E., Everdingen, J. J., Huijsman, R., & Grol, R. P. (2008). Evidence for the impact of quality improvement collaboratives: Systematic review. *British Medical Journal, 336*(7659), 1491–1494.

Schuster, M. A., McGlynn, E. A., & Brook, R. H. (1998). How good is the quality of healthcare in the United States? *Milbank Quarterly, 83,* 843–895.

Slade, S. C., Kent, P., Patel, S., Bucknall, T., & Buchbinder, R. (2016). Barriers to primary care clinician adherence to clinical guidelines for the management of low back pain: A systematic review and metasynthesis of qualitative studies. *Clinical Journal of Pain, 32*(9), 800–816.

Wade, D. T., & Halligan, P. W. (2004). Do biomedical models of illness make for good healthcare systems? *British Medical Journal, 329*(7479), 1398–1401.

Wåhlin, C., Ekberg, K., Persson, J., Bernfort, L., & Öberg, B. (2012). Association between clinical and work-related interventions and return-to-work for patients with musculoskeletal or mental disorders. *Journal of Rehabilitation Medicine, 44,* 355–362.

Walker, M. J., Boyles, R. E., Young, B. A., Strunce, J. B., Garber, M. B., Whitman, J. M., . . . Wainner, R. S. (2008). The effectiveness of manual physical therapy and exercise for mechanical neck pain: A randomized clinical trial. *Spine, 33*(22), 2371–2378.

Webster, B. S., Bauer, A. Z., Choi, Y., Cifuentes, M., & Pransky, G. S. (2013). Iatrogenic consequences of early magnetic resonance imaging in acute, work-related, disabling low back pain. *Spine, 38*(22), 1939–1946.

INDEX